# Cardiopulmonary Bypass

D1557463

# Cardiopulmonary Bypass

Edited by

**Sunit Ghosh**

**Florian Falter**

**David J. Cook**

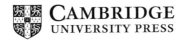

CAMBRIDGE UNIVERSITY PRESS
Cambridge, New York, Melbourne, Madrid, Cape Town, Singapore,
São Paulo, Delhi, Dubai, Tokyo

Cambridge University Press
The Edinburgh Building, Cambridge CB2 8RU, UK

Published in the United States of America by
Cambridge University Press, New York

www.cambridge.org
Information on this title: www.cambridge.org/9780521721998

First published 2009

Printed in the United Kingdom at the University Press, Cambridge

A catalog record for this publication is available from the
British Library

ISBN 978-0-521-72199-8 Paperback

Additional resources for this publication at
www.cambridge.org/9780521721998

# Contents

*List of contributors* vii
*Preface* ix

1. **Equipment and monitoring** 1
   Victoria Chilton and Andrew Klein

2. **Circuit setup and safety checks** 23
   Simon Colah and Steve Gray

3. **Priming solutions for cardiopulmonary bypass circuits** 36
   George Hallward and Roger Hall

4. **Anticoagulation, coagulopathies, blood transfusion and conservation** 41
   Liza Enriquez and Linda Shore-Lesserson

5. **Conduct of cardiopulmonary bypass** 54
   Betsy Evans, Helen Dunningham and John Wallwork

6. **Metabolic management during cardiopulmonary bypass** 70
   Kevin Collins and G. Burkhard Mackensen

7. **Myocardial protection and cardioplegia** 80
   Constantine Athanasuleas and Gerald D. Buckberg

8. **Weaning from cardiopulmonary bypass** 92
   James Keogh, Susanna Price and Brian Keogh

9. **Mechanical circulatory support** 106
   Kirsty Dempster and Steven Tsui

10. **Deep hypothermic circulatory arrest** 125
    Joe Arrowsmith and Charles W. Hogue

11. **Organ damage during cardiopulmonary bypass** 140
    Andrew Snell and Barbora Parizkova

12. **Cerebral morbidity in adult cardiac surgery** 153
    David Cook

13. **Acute kidney injury (AKI)** 167
    Robert C. Albright

14. **Extracorporeal membrane oxygenation** 176
    Ashish A. Bartakke and Giles J. Peek

15. **Cardiopulmonary bypass in non-cardiac procedures** 187
    Sukumaran Nair

*Index* 199

# Contributors

**Robert C. Albright Jr DO**
Assistant Professor of Medicine, Division of Nephrology and Hypertension, Mayo Clinic, Rochester, Minnesota, USA

**Joe Arrowsmith MD FRCP FRCA**
Consultant Cardiothoracic Anaesthetist, Papworth Hospital, Cambridge, UK

**Constantine Athanasuleas MD**
Division of Cardiothoracic Surgery, University of Alabama, Birmingham, Alabama, USA

**Ashish A Bartakke MD (Anaesthesia), MBBS**
ECMO Research Fellow, Glenfield Hospital, Leicester, UK

**Gerald D. Buckberg MD**
Distinguished Professor of Surgery, Department of Cardiothoracic Surgery, David Geffen School of Medicine at UCLA, Los Angeles, California, USA

**Victoria Chilton BSc CCP**
Senior Clinical Perfusion Scientist, Alder Hey Children's Hospital, Liverpool, UK

**Simon Colah MSc FCP CCP**
Senior Clinical Perfusion Scientist, Cambridge Perfusion Services, Cambridge, UK

**Kevin Collins BSN CCP LP**
Staff Perfusionist, Duke University Medical Center, Durham, North Carolina, USA

**David Cook MD**
Associate Professor, Department of Anesthesiology, Mayo Clinic, Rochester, Minnesota, USA

**Kirsty Dempster CCP**
Senior Clinical Perfusion Scientist, Cambridge Perfusion Services, Cambridge, UK

**Helen Dunningham BSc CCP**
Senior Clinical Perfusion Scientist, Cambridge Perfusion Services, Cambridge, UK

**Liza Enriquez MD**
Fellow, Department of Anesthesiology, Montefiore Medical Center, Albert Einstein College of Medicine, New York, USA

**Betsy Evans MA MRCS**
Registrar in Cardiothoracic Surgery, Papworth Hospital, Cambridge, UK

**Steve Gray MBBS FRCA**
Consultant Cardiothoracic Anaesthetist, Papworth Hospital, Cambridge, UK

**Roger Hall MBChB FANZCA FRCA**
Consultant Cardiothoracic Anaesthetist, Papworth Hospital, Cambridge, UK

**George Hallward MBBS MRCP FRCA**
Clinical Fellow in Cardiothoracic Anaesthesia, Papworth Hospital, Cambridge, UK

**Charles W. Hogue MD**
Associate Professor of Anesthesiology and Critical Care Medicine, The Johns Hopkins Medical Institutions and The Johns Hopkins Hospital, Baltimore, Maryland, USA

**Brian Keogh MBBS FRCA**
Consultant Anaesthetist, Royal Brompton & Harefield NHS Trust, UK

**James Keogh MBChB FRCA**
Clinical Fellow in Paediatric Cardiothoracic Anaesthesia, Royal Brompton & Harefield NHS Trust, UK

**Andrew Klein MBBS FRCA**
Consultant Cardiothoracic Anaesthetist, Papworth Hospital, Cambridge, UK

**G. Burkhard Mackensen MD PhD FASE**
Associate Professor, Department of Anesthesiology, Duke University Medical Center, Durham, North Carolina, USA

**Sukumaran Nair MBBS FRCS**
Consultant Cardiothoracic Surgeon, Papworth Hospital, Cambridge, UK

**Barbora Parizkova MD**
Clinical Fellow in Cardiothoracic Anaesthesia, Papworth Hospital, Cambridge, UK

**Giles J Peek MD FRCS**
Consultant in Cardiothoracic Surgery & ECMO, Glenfield Hospital, Leicester, UK

**Susanna Price MBBS BSc MRCP EDICM PhD**
Consultant Cardiologist and Intensivist, Royal Brompton & Harefield NHS Trust, UK

**Linda Shore-Lesserson MD**
Professor, Department of Anesthesiology, Montefiore Medical Center, Albert Einstein College of Medicine, New York, USA

**Andrew Snell MBChB, FANZCA**
Clinical Fellow in Cardiothoracic Anaesthesia, Papworth Hospital, Cambridge, UK

**Steven Tsui MBBCh FRCS**
Consultant in Cardiothoracic Surgery/Director of Transplant Services, Papworth Hospital, Cambridge, UK

**John Wallwork MA MBBCh FRCS FRCP**
Professor, Department of Cardiothoracic Surgery, Papworth Hospital, Cambridge, UK

# Preface

This book has been written to provide an easily readable source of material for the everyday practice of clinical perfusion. For the past few years there has been a dearth of books, other than large reference tomes, relating to cardiopulmonary bypass. We hope that newcomers to the subject will find this book useful, both in the clinical setting and in preparation for examinations, and that more experienced perfusionists and medical staff will find it useful for preparing teaching material or for guidance.

We would like to thank everyone who helped in the preparation of the manuscript, particularly those who contributed their expertise by writing chapters for this book.

*S. Ghosh, F. Falter and D. J. Cook*

# Equipment and monitoring

Victoria Chilton and Andrew Klein

The optimum conditions for cardiothoracic surgery have traditionally been regarded as a "still and bloodless" surgical field. Cardiopulmonary bypass (CPB) provides this by incorporating a pump to substitute for the function of the heart and a gas exchange device, the "oxygenator," to act as an artificial lung. Cardiopulmonary bypass thus allows the patient's heart and lungs to be temporarily devoid of circulation, and respiratory and cardiac activity suspended, so that intricate cardiac, vascular or thoracic surgery can be performed in a safe and controlled environment.

## History

In its most basic form, the CPB machine and circuit comprises of plastic tubing, a reservoir, an oxygenator and a pump. Venous blood is drained by gravity into the reservoir via a cannula placed in the right atrium or a large vein, pumped through the oxygenator and returned into the patient's arterial system via a cannula in the aorta or other large artery. Transit through the oxygenator reduces the partial pressure of carbon dioxide in the blood and raises oxygen content. A typical CPB circuit is shown in Figure 1.1.

Cardiac surgery has widely been regarded as one of the most important medical advances of the twentieth century. The concept of a CPB machine arose from the technique of "cross-circulation" in which the arterial and venous circulations of mother and child were connected by tubing in series. The mother's heart and lungs maintained the circulatory and respiratory functions of both, whilst surgeons operated on the child's heart (Dr Walton Lillehei, Minnesota, 1953, see Figure 1.2a). Modern CPB machines (see Figure 1.2b) have evolved to incorporate monitoring and safety features in their design.

John Gibbon (Philadelphia, 1953) is credited with developing the first mechanical CPB system, which he used when repairing an atrial secundum defect (ASD). Initially, the technology was complex and unreliable and was therefore slow to develop. The equipment used in a typical extracorporeal circuit has advanced rapidly since this time and although circuits vary considerably among surgeons and hospitals, the basic concepts are essentially common to all CPB circuits.

This chapter describes the standard equipment and monitoring components of the CPB machine and extracorporeal circuit as well as additional equipment such as the suckers used to scavenge blood from the operative field, cardioplegia delivery systems and hemofilters (see Tables 1.1 and 1.2).

## Tubing

The tubing in the CPB circuit interconnects all of the main components of the circuit. A variety of materials may be used for the manufacture of the tubing; these include polyvinyl chloride

*Cardiopulmonary Bypass*, ed. S. Ghosh, F. Falter and D. J. Cook. Published by Cambridge University Press.
© Cambridge University Press 2009.

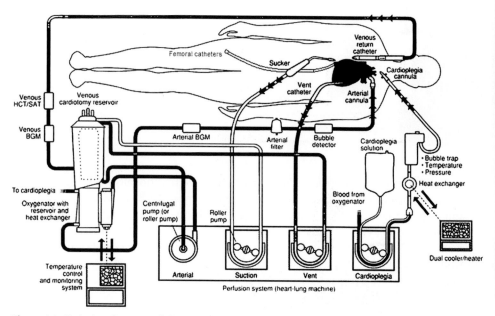

**Figure 1.1.** Typical configuration of a basic cardiopulmonary bypass circuit. BGM = blood gas monitor; SAT = oxygen saturation.

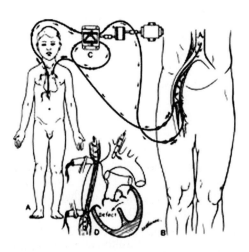

**Figure 1.2a.** Depiction of the method of direct vision intracardiac surgery utilizing extracorporeal circulation by means of controlled cross circulation. The patient (A), showing sites of arterial and venous cannulations. The donor (B), showing sites of arterial and venous (superficial femoral and great saphenous) cannulations. The Sigma motor pump (C) controlling precisely the reciprocal exchange of blood between the patient and donor. Close-up of the patient's heart (D), showing the vena caval catheter positioned to draw venous blood from both the superior and inferior venae cavae during the cardiac bypass interval. The arterial blood from the donor circulated to the patient's body through the catheter that was inserted into the left subclavian artery. (Reproduced with kind permission from Lillehei CW, Cohen M, Warden HE, *et al.* The results of direct vision closure of ventricular septal defects in eight patients by means of controlled cross circulation. Surg Gynecol Obstet 1955; 101: 446. Copyright American College of Surgeons.)

(PVC, by far the most commonly used), silicone (reserved for the arterial pump boot) and latex rubber. The size of tubing used at different points in the circuit is determined by the pressure and rate of blood flow that will be required through that region of the circuit, or through a particular component of the circuit (see Table 1.3).

PVC is made up of polymer chains with polar carbon-chloride (C-Cl) bonds. These bonds result in considerable intermolecular attraction between the polymer chains, making PVC a fairly strong material. The feature of PVC that accounts for its widespread use is its versatility. On its own, PVC is a fairly rigid plastic, but plasticizers can be added to make it highly flexible. Plasticizers are molecules that incorporate between the polymer chains allowing them

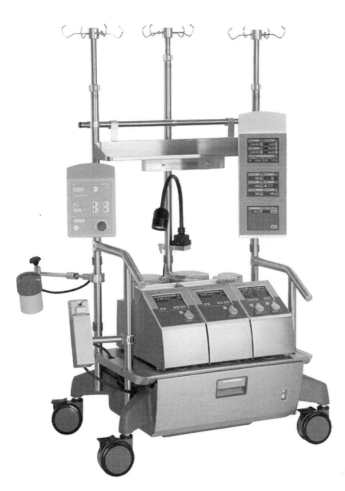

**Figure 1.2b.** Cardiopulmonary bypass machine (reproduced with kind permission of Sorin Group).

to slide over one another more easily, thus increasing the flexibility of the PVC. However, one disadvantage is that PVC tubing stiffens during hypothermic CPB and tends to induce spallation; that is, the release of plastic microparticles from the inner wall of tubing as a result of pump compressions.

Other materials used to manufacture perfusion tubing include latex rubber and silicone rubber. Latex rubber generates more hemolysis than PVC, whereas silicone rubber is known to produce less hemolysis when the pump is completely occluded, but can release more particles than PVC. As a result of this, and because of PVC's durability and accepted hemolysis rates, PVC is the most widely used tubing material. The arterial roller pump boot is the main exception to this, as the tubing at this site is constantly compressed by the rollers themselves, leading to the use of silicone tubing for this purpose.

## Arterial cannulae

The arterial cannula is used to connect the "arterial limb" of the CPB circuit to the patient and so deliver oxygenated blood from the heart-lung machine directly into the patient's arterial system. The required size is determined by the size of the vessel that is being cannulated,

**Table 1.1.** Components of the CPB machine and the extracorporeal circuit

| Equipment | Function |
|---|---|
| Oxygenator system, venous reservoir, oxygenator, heat exchanger | Oxygenate, remove carbon dioxide and cool/re-warm blood |
| Gas line and FiO$_2$ blender | Delivers fresh gas to the oxygenator in a controlled mixture |
| Arterial pump | Pumps blood at a set flow rate to the patient |
| Cardiotomy suckers and vents | Scavenges blood from the operative field and vents the heart |
| Arterial line filter | Removes microaggregates and particulate matter >40 μm |
| Cardioplegia systems | Deliver high-dose potassium solutions to arrest the heart and preserve the myocardium |
| Cannulae | Connect the patient to the extracorporeal circuit |

**Table 1.2.** Monitoring components of the CPB machine and the extracorporeal circuit

| Monitoring device | Function |
|---|---|
| Low-level alarm | Alarms when level in the reservoir reaches minimum running volume |
| Pressure monitoring (line pressure, blood cardioplegia pressure and vent pressure) | Alarms when line pressure exceeds set limits |
| Bubble detector (arterial line and blood cardioplegia) | Alarms when bubbles are sensed |
| Oxygen sensor | Alarms when oxygen supply to the oxygenator fails |
| S$_a$O$_2$, S$_v$O$_2$, and hemoglobin monitor | Continuously measures these levels from the extracorporeal circuit |
| In-line blood gas monitoring | Continuously measures arterial and venous gases from the extracorporeal circuit |
| Perfusionist | Constantly monitors the cardiopulmonary bypass machine and the extracorporeal circuit |

**Table 1.3.** Tubing sizes commonly used in different parts of the extracorporeal circuit (adults only)

| Tubing size | Function |
|---|---|
| 3/16″ (4.5 mm) | Cardioplegia section of the blood cardioplegia delivery system |
| 1/4″ (6.0 mm) | Suction tubing, blood section of the blood cardioplegia delivery system |
| 3/8″ (9.0 mm) | Arterial pump line for flow rates <6.7 l/minute, majority of the arterial tubing in the extracorporeal circuit |
| 1/2″ (12.0 mm) | Venous line, larger tubing is required to gravity drain blood from the patient |

as well as the blood flow required. The ascending aorta is the most common site of arterial cannulation for routine cardiovascular surgery. This is because the ascending aorta is readily accessible for cannulation when a median sternotomy approach is used and has the lowest associated incidence of aortic dissection (0.01–0.09%). After sternotomy and exposure, the surgeon is able to assess the size of the aorta before choosing the most appropriately sized cannula (see Table 1.4).

**Table 1.4.** Arterial cannulae flow rates in relation to type/size

| Cannulae | Size | | Flow rate (l/minute) |
|---|---|---|---|
| | French gauge | mm | |
| DLP angled tip | 20 | 6.7 | 6.5 |
| | 22 | 7.3 | 8.0 |
| | 24 | 8.0 | 9.0 |
| DLD straight tip | 21 | 7.0 | 5.0 |
| | 24 | 8.0 | 6.0 |
| Sarns high flow angled tip | 15.6 | 5.2 | 3.5 |
| | 19.5 | 6.5 | 5.25 |
| | 24 | 8.0 | 8.0 |
| Sarns straight tip | 20 | 6.7 | 5.9 |
| | 22 | 7.3 | 6.0 |
| | 24 | 8.0 | 6.0 |

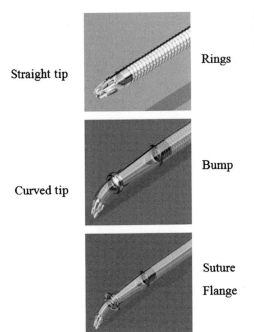

Straight tip — Rings

Curved tip — Bump

Suture
Flange

**Figure 1.3.** Commonly used arterial cannulae. (Reproduced with kind permission from Edwards Lifesciences.)

Thin-walled cannulae are preferred, as they present lower resistance to flow because of their larger effective internal diameter. This leads to a reduction in arterial line pressure within the extracorporeal circuit and increased blood flow to the patient.

Arterial cannulae with an angled tip are available. These direct blood flow towards the aortic arch rather than towards the wall of the aorta; this may minimize damage to the vessel wall. In addition, cannulae with a flange near the tip to aid secure fixation to the vessel wall and cannulae that incorporate a spirally wound wire within their wall to prevent "kinking" and obstruction are commonly used (see Figure 1.3).

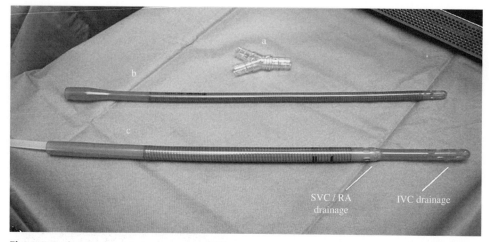

SVC / RA
drainage

IVC drainage

**Figure 1.4.** Commonly used venous cannulae: (a) Y-connector to connect single-stage cannulae; (b) single-stage cannula; (c) two-stage cannula. RA, right atrial; SVC, superior vena cava; IVC, inferior vena cava.

## Venous cannulae

Venous cannulation for CPB allows deoxygenated blood to be drained from the patient into the extracorporeal circuit. The type of venous cannulation used is dependent upon the operation being undertaken. For cardiac surgery that does not involve opening the chambers of the heart, for example, coronary artery bypass grafts (CABG), a two-stage venous cannula is often used. The distal portion, i.e., the tip of the cannula, sits in the inferior vena cava (IVC) and drains blood from the IVC through holes around the tip. A second series of holes in the cannula, a few centimeters above the tip, is sited in the right atrium, to drain venous blood entering the atrium via the superior vena cava (SVC).

An alternative method of venous cannulation for CPB is bicaval cannulation – this uses two single-stage cannulae that sit in the inferior and superior vena cavae, respectively. The two single-stage cannulae are connected using a Y-connector to the venous line of the CPB circuit. Bicaval cannulation is generally used for procedures that require the cardiac chambers to be opened, as the two separate pipes in the IVC and SVC permit unobstructed venous drainage during surgical manipulation of the dissected heart and keep the heart completely empty of blood (see Figure 1.4).

The femoral veins may also be used as a cannulation site for more complex surgery. In this instance, a long cannula, which is in essence an elongated single-stage cannula, may be passed up the femoral vein into the vena cava in order to achieve venous drainage.

As with arterial cannulation, the size of the cannulae will depend on the vessels being cannulated as well as the desired blood flow. It is important to use appropriately sized cannulae in order to obtain maximum venous drainage from the patient so that full flow can be achieved when CPB is commenced.

## Pump heads

There are two types of pumps used in extracorporeal circuits:
1. Those that produce a flow – roller pumps.
2. Those that produce a pressure – centrifugal pumps.

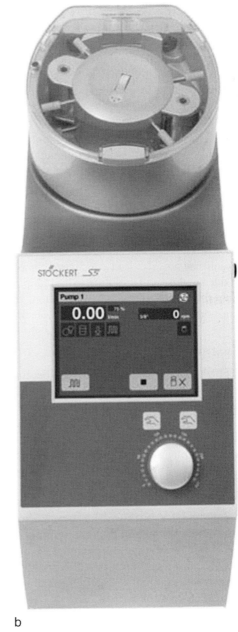

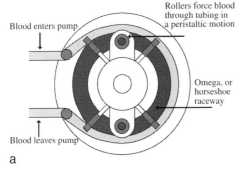

a           b

**Figure 1.5.** (a) Line drawing of a roller pump; (b) a roller pump. (Reproduced with kind permission from Sorin Group.)

## Roller pumps

Initial technology developed in the mid twentieth century used non-pulsatile roller pumps in CPB machines. This technology has not changed greatly over the past 50 years.

Roller pumps positively displace blood through the tubing using a peristaltic motion. Two rollers, opposite each other, "roll" the blood through the tubing. When the tubing is intermittently occluded, positive and negative pressures are generated on either side of the point of occlusion. Forward or retrograde flow of blood can be achieved by altering the direction of pump head rotation; thus roller pumps are commonly used as the primary arterial flow pump as well as for suction of blood from the heart and mediastinal cavity during CPB to salvage blood. Roller pumps are relatively independent of circuit resistance and hydrostatic pressure; output depends on the number of rotations of the pump head and the internal diameter of the tubing used (see Figure 1.5a,b).

This type of positive displacement pump can be set to provide pulsatile or non-pulsatile (laminar) flow. Debate over the advantages and disadvantages of non-pulsatile or pulsatile perfusion during cardiopulmonary bypass still continues. Non-pulsatile perfusion is known to have a detrimental effect on cell metabolism and organ function. The main argument in favor of pulsatile perfusion is that it more closely resembles the pattern of blood flow generated by the cardiac cycle and should therefore more closely emulate the flow characteristics of the physiological circulation, particularly enhancing flow through smaller capillary networks in comparison to non-pulsatile perfusion. The increased shear stress from the changing positive and negative pressures generated to aid pulsatile perfusion may, however, lead to increased hemolysis. Roller pumps have one further disadvantage: sudden occlusion of the inflow to the pump, as a result of low circulating volume or venous cannula obstruction, can result in "cavitation," the formation and collapse of gas bubbles due to the creation of pockets of low pressure by precipitous change in mechanical forces.

## Centrifugal pumps

In 1973, the Biomedicus model 600 became the first disposable centrifugal pump head for clinical use. The Biomedicus head contains a cone with a metal bearing encased in an outer housing, forming a sealed unit through which blood can flow. When in use the head is seated on a pump drive unit. The cone spins as a result of the magnetic force that is generated when the pump is activated. The spinning cone creates a negative pressure that sucks blood into the inlet, creating a vortex. Centrifugal force imparts kinetic energy on the blood as the pump spins at 2000–4000 rpm (this speed is set by the user). The energy created in the cone creates pressure and blood is then forced out of the outlet. The resulting blood flow will depend on the pressure gradient and the resistance at the outlet of the pump (a combination of the CPB circuit and the systemic vascular resistance of the patient). Flow meters are included in all centrifugal pumps and rely on ultrasonic or electromagnetic principles to determine blood flow velocity accurately (see Figure 1.6a–c).

Despite extensive research, there is little evidence to show any benefit of one type of pump over another in clinical practice. Centrifugal pumps may produce less hemolysis and platelet activation than roller pumps, but this does not correlate with any difference in clinical outcome, including neurological function. They are certainly more expensive (as the pump head is single use) and may be prone to heat generation and clot formation on the rotating surfaces in contact with blood. In general, they are reserved for more complex surgery of prolonged duration, during which the damage to blood components associated with roller pumps may be theoretically disadvantageous.

## Reservoirs

Cardiotomy reservoirs may be hardshell or collapsible. Hardshell reservoirs are most commonly used in adult cardiac surgery; collapsible reservoirs are still used by some institutions

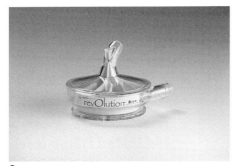

a

**Figure 1.6.** (a) Centrifugal pump. (b) Schematic diagram of centrifugal pump. (c) Schematic cut through centrifugal pump. (a, b Reproduced with kind permission from Sorin Group.)

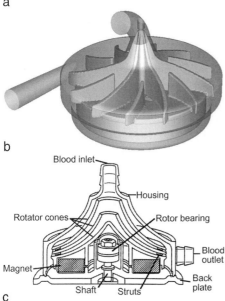

b

c

for pediatric and adult cases. Hardshell reservoirs usually comprise of a polycarbonate housing, a polyester depth filter and a polyurethane de-foamer. The reservoir component of the CPB circuit therefore provides high-efficiency filtration, de-foaming and the removal of foreign particles (see Figure 1.7).

The reservoir acts as a chamber for the venous blood to drain into before it is pumped into the oxygenator and permits ready access for the addition of fluids and drugs. A level of fluid is maintained in the reservoir for the duration of CPB. This reduces the risks of perfusion accidents, such as pumping large volumes of air into the arterial circulation if the venous return to the CPB machine from the patient is occluded for any reason.

Blood that is scavenged from the operative field via the suckers is returned to the reservoir. The salvaged blood is mixed with air and may contain tissue debris. It is therefore vital for this blood to be filtered through the reservoir before being pumped to the patient. The reservoir is constantly vented to prevent the pressure build-up that could occur if the suckers were left running at a high level for the duration of the procedure. The salvaged blood from the vents that the surgeon uses to prevent the heart from distending during CPB also returns to the reservoir.

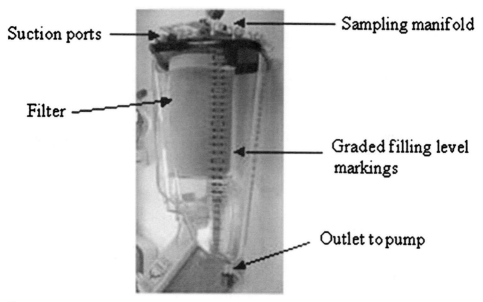

Suction ports —→

Sampling manifold

Filter —→

Graded filling level markings

Outlet to pump

**Figure 1.7.** Reservoir in CPB circuit.

## Oxygenators

The present success of cardiac surgery relies heavily on extracorporeal perfusion techniques employing an efficient gas exchange mechanism: the oxygenator. The requirements of the oxygenator include efficient oxygenation of desaturated hemoglobin and simultaneous removal of carbon dioxide from the blood. The oxygenator therefore acts as an artificial alveolar-pulmonary capillary system.

Gas exchange is based on Fick's Law of Diffusion:

$$\text{Volume of Gas diffused} = \frac{\text{Diffusion coefficient} \times \text{Partial pressure difference}}{\text{Distance to travel}}$$

The oxygenator provides an interface of high surface area between blood on one side and gas on the other. The distance gas has to travel across the interface is minimized by constructing the membrane from very thin material.

In the early 1950s, attempts were made to oxygenate the blood using techniques such as cross circulation between related humans, or using animal lungs for patients undergoing open heart surgery. In 1955, DeWall and Lillehei devised the first helical reservoir to be used; this was an early form of the bubble oxygenator. One year later, in 1956, the rotating disc oxygenator was developed. In 1966, DeWall introduced the hardshell bubble oxygenator with integral heat exchanger. Subsequently, Lillehei and Lande developed a commercially manufactured, disposable, compact membrane oxygenator.

Currently, most commonly used oxygenators are membrane oxygenators with a microporous polypropylene hollow fiber structure. The membrane is initially porous, but proteins in blood rapidly coat it, preventing direct blood/gas contact. The surface tension of the blood also prevents plasma water from entering the gas phase of the micropores during CPB and prevents gas leakage into the blood phase, thus reducing microemboli. However, after several hours of use, evaporation and condensation of serum leaking through micropores leads to

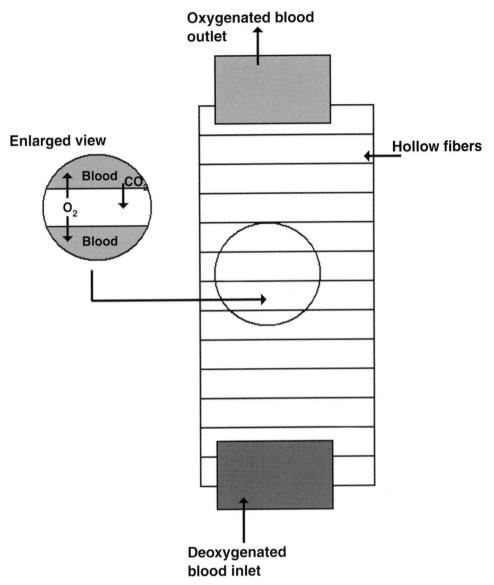

**Figure 1.8.** Schematic cut through an oxygenator.

reduced efficiency and therefore the majority of these types of oxygenators must be changed after about 6 hours.

The majority of oxygenators consist of a module for gas exchange with an integrated heat exchanger. An external heater–cooler pumps temperature-controlled water into the heat exchanger, which is separated from the blood by a highly thermally conductive material. This is biologically inert, to reduce the risk of blood component activation. The external heater–cooler has digital regulating modules to allow precise control of temperature through thermostat-controlled heating and cooling elements within the console. Controlled cooling and re-warming of the patient are crucial to ensure an even distribution of

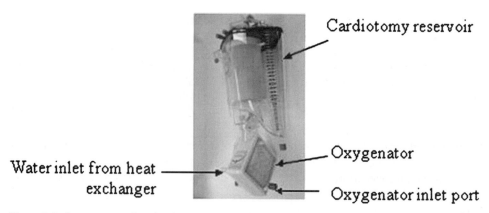

**Figure 1.9.** Oxygenator combined with a reservoir and a heat exchanger in a single unit.

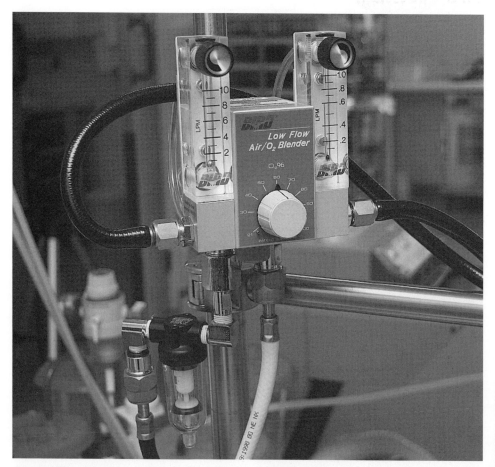

**Figure 1.10** Rotameters on a CPB machine to regulate sweep gas flow.

temperature throughout the body and to prevent damage to blood components, proteins and tissues.

The Cobe Duo (Cobe Cardiovascular CML-Duo) adult cardiovascular membrane oxygenator comprises of a microporous polypropylene pleated sheet that has a prime volume of approximately 250 ml and works on the principle of diffusion. Blood first passes over an integral heat exchanger, changes temperature and then moves into the oxygenator compartment. Gas supplies of oxygen, air and carbon dioxide are delivered to the membrane in controlled quantities. This "sweep" gas flows inside the fibers and has a higher concentration of oxygen than venous blood on the outside of the fibers, enabling oxygen to move along a concentration gradient across the membrane into the blood to create equilibrium. Carbon dioxide, which is present in a high concentration in the venous blood, moves in the opposite direction, across the membrane into the gas phase (see Figures 1.8 and 1.9). The exhaust gases are scavenged from outlet ports on the back of the oxygenator.

## Gas supply system

The gas supply system provides a source of oxygen, air and carbon dioxide to the oxygenator. A blender mixes piped oxygen and air to the concentration set by the user, and the gas is delivered at a rate set on a flow meter (see Figure 1.10). Flow meters may be digital or mechanical rotameters. An oxygen analyzer is included in the gas circuit to continuously display the concentration of oxygen delivered in order to prevent the inadvertent administration of a hypoxic mixture. An anesthetic vaporizer may be incorporated, along with a means of scavenging waste gases.

## Filters and bubble traps

There are numerous filters that can be used within the extracorporeal circuit. These range from 0.2 μm gas line filters to 40 μm arterial line filters (see Table 1.5).

**Table 1.5.** Filtration devices used within the cardiopulmonary bypass circuit

| Filter type | Application and specification |
|---|---|
| Gas line | Removes 99.999% of bacteria found in the gas stream minimizing cross-contamination between the patient and the equipment |
| Pre-CPB | 0.2 μm filter is used during the priming and re-circulation phase. It is designed for the removal of inadvertent particulate debris and microbial contaminants and their associated endotoxins |
| Arterial line | Designed to remove microemboli >40 μm in size from the perfusate during extracorporeal circulation. This includes gas emboli, fat emboli and aggregates composed of platelets, red blood cells and other debris |
| Leukodepletion | Reduces the levels of leukocytes, either from the arterial line or cardioplegia system, and excludes microemboli >40 μm |
| Cardioplegia | Blood cardioplegia: >40 μm filter. Crystalloid cardioplegia: >0.2 μm filter. Low priming volume filter for cell-free solutions. Removes inadvertent particulate debris and microbial contaminants and their associated endotoxins |
| Blood transfusion | Designed to reduce the levels of leukocytes and microaggregates from 1 unit of packed red blood cells or whole blood |
| Cell salvage | Designed for the filtration of salvaged blood to remove potentially harmful microaggregates, leukocytes and lipid particles |

Adapted from Pall product specifications 2007.

**Table 1.6.** Different commercially available arterial line filters

| Manufacturer | Filter type | Fiber material | Filter size (μm) |
| --- | --- | --- | --- |
| Bentley | Screen | Heparin-coated polyester | 25 |
| Delta | Screen | Nylon | 40 |
| Lifeline-Delhi | Screen | Unspecified | 40 |
| Pall | Screen | Heparin-coated polyester | 40 |
| Swank | Depth | Dacron wool | 13 |

Arterial line filters are the most commonly used additional filtration devices. They are indicated for use in all CPB procedures and there are a number of filters available with slightly different characteristics (see Table 1.6).

Screen filters remove particles by mechanical retention and impaction. They have a specific pore size and remove air by velocity separation and venting. Swank is the only manufacturer of depth filters at present. This type of filter creates a tortuous path between fibers and retains particles mechanically. There is not normally a specific pore size. Air is removed by entrapment during transit of blood through the pathway between fibers.

The US Food and Drug Administration (FDA) have outlined key areas of importance pertaining to arterial line filters (FDA, 2000). These are summarized as follows:

- amount of damage to formed blood elements, for example, clotting and hemolysis;
- degree of pressure drop resulting in inadequate blood flow, damage to the device, structural integrity and damage to the arterial line;
- structural integrity of the product;
- excessive pressure gradients, for example, blood damage and inadequate blood flow;
- filtration efficiency and gas emboli-handling capacities;
- user error;
- blood incompatibility and the requirements of ISO 10993: Biological Evaluation of Medical Devices;
- compatibility of the product when exposed to circulating blood and infections; and
- shelf life.

These stringent criteria aim to ensure the production of high-quality arterial line filters that will not have any deleterious effects on the CPB circuit or patient.

## Suckers and vents

The suckers attached to the CPB circuit allow blood to be salvaged from the operative field to be returned to the circuit via the reservoir.

"Vent" suckers are specifically used to drain blood that has not been directly removed from the heart by the venous pipes. The most common sites for placing dedicated vents are:

- the aortic root;
- the left ventricle;
- the right superior pulmonary vein;
- the left ventricular apex; and
- the left atrium or pulmonary artery.

There are a number of reasons for venting the heart during CPB:

- to prevent distension of the heart;
- to reduce myocardial re-warming;
- to evacuate air from the cardiac chambers during the de-airing phase of the procedure;
- to improve surgical exposure; and
- to create a dry surgical field, especially during the distal coronary anastamosis phase of CABG surgery.

There are complications associated with all sites used for venting, most commonly relating to injury to tissues at the site. Venting via the left ventricular (LV) apex, however, is associated with particularly serious consequences including:

- damage to the LV wall due to excessive suction;
- LV wall rupture if inadequately closed at the end of the bypass period; and
- embolization through air entrained into the LV.

Active venting with high levels of suction can lead to air being introduced into the arterial side of the CPB circuit due to a small percentage of air sucked into the venous side of the reservoir and oxygenator passing through the circuit into the arterial side. Therefore, suction pressure and duration should be kept to a minimum.

# Cardioplegia delivery systems

One of the major concerns during cardiac surgery is protection of the heart during the operation. Myocardial protection is discussed more fully in Chapter 7. During the period in which the heart is devoid of blood supply, the myocardial cells continue to utilize high-energy phosphates (adenosine triphosphate, ATP) to fuel metabolic reactions anaerobically. This results in depletion of energy reserves and the build up of products of anaerobic metabolism, such as lactic acid. These processes decrease myocardial contractility in the period immediately following restoration of blood flow and myocardial function remains compromised until ATP reserves are restored and the products of anaerobic metabolism decline in concentration. Preservation of myocardial function during the ischemic period, that is, during the period in which the aorta is cross-clamped, is best achieved by putting the heart into a state of hibernation using a solution – generically termed "cardioplegia." The purpose of cardioplegia is to cause rapid diastolic cardiac arrest. This produces a still, flaccid heart, which facilitates surgery and also is the state in which myocardial metabolism is almost at its lowest levels. Further reduction in the metabolic state of the heart is achieved by cooling using cold cardioplegia and also by core cooling of the body.

The common constituent of all cardioplegia solutions is a high concentration of potassium, as this produces diastolic cardiac arrest. The other constituents of cardioplegia vary widely from normal saline solution to blood mixed with complex antioxidants. The delivery of cardioplegia may be as a single bolus, intermittent boluses or continuous infusion or combinations of all three. The administration techniques have progressed from un-monitored pressurized delivery into the root of the aorta; current practice is discussed more fully in Chapter 7. The delivery sites for the cardioplegia vary according to surgical preference and the operation being performed and include: directly into the aortic root, the coronary ostia, the saphenous vein graft or retrograde via the coronary sinus. The flow rates and pressures that the cardioplegia solution is delivered at will vary depending on the mode of delivery.

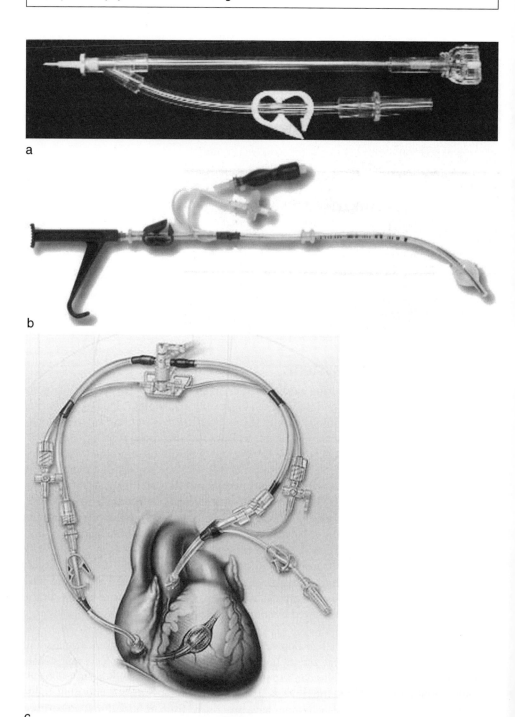

**Figure 1.11** (a) Double-lumen aortic root cannula, which can be used to deliver cardioplegia and as an aortic root vent. (b) Retrograde cardioplegia delivery cannula. (c) Schematic drawing of antegrade and retrograde cardioplegia delivery. (Reproduced with kind permission from Edwards Lifesciences.)

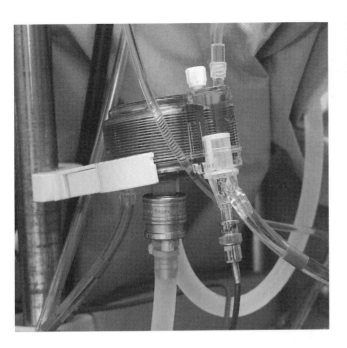

**Figure 1.12** Cardioplegia delivery system: allows mixing of blood and cardioplegia solution and warming or cooling of solution before application.

**Table 1.7.** Cardioplegia delivery systems

| Manufacturer | Integrated heat exchanger | Air trap removal | Delivery system |
|---|---|---|---|
| Sorin | Yes | Yes | Blood cardioplegia 4:1 ratio via roller pump |
| Medtronic | Yes | Yes | Blood cardioplegia 4:1 ratio via roller pump (can also be used with a syringe driver for the potassium solutions) |
| Lifeline-Delhi | Yes | Yes | Blood cardioplegia 4:1 ratio via a roller pump |
| Aeon Medical | Yes | Yes | Blood cardioplegia 4:1 ratio via a roller pump |

Different types of cannulae are available for delivery of cardioplegia via the various sites (see Figure 1.11).

Many different designs of cardioplegia delivery systems are available (see Figure 1.12). Almost all of the systems allow delivery of warm and cold solutions and allow the mixing of crystalloid solutions with blood (see Table 1.7). The systems also allow the monitoring of the cardioplegia infusion line pressure. This is essential when delivering cardioplegia into small vessels and the coronary sinus to prevent damage.

# Hemofilters

Also known as ultrafilters or hemoconcentrators, these contain semipermeable membranes (hollow fibers) that permit passage of water and electrolytes out of blood. They are normally

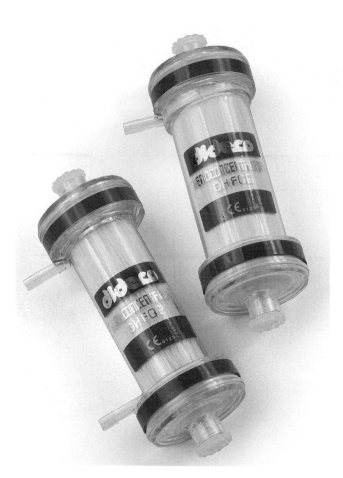

**Figure 1.13** Hemofilters. (Reproduced with kind permission from Sorin Group.)

connected to the CPB circuit at a high pressure port or line, such as the systemic flow line, to provide a driving force for blood through the device. This allows blood to be filtered before being returned to the patient. Fluid removal is usually 30 to 50 ml/minute, and depending on the membrane used, molecules of up to 20 000 Daltons are removed. Hemofiltration may be used during or after CPB, mainly to manage hyperkalemia or acidosis, but also to concentrate the blood if the hematocrit (HCT) is low and circulating volume is adequate (see Figure 1.13).

## Monitoring

Extracorporeal perfusion techniques require a large amount of vigilance from the entire team involved in the patient's care. Setup and safety features during CPB are discussed in more detail in Chapter 2.

## In-line blood gas analysis and venous saturation/hematocrit monitors

The theoretical advantages of using continuous in-line blood gas and electrolyte monitoring during CPB are well established; however, the clinical impact remains controversial. These devices may be divided into those using electrochemical electrodes and cuvettes, which are placed in the circuit, and those that use light absorbance or reflectance, which require sensors placed external to the circuit tubing.

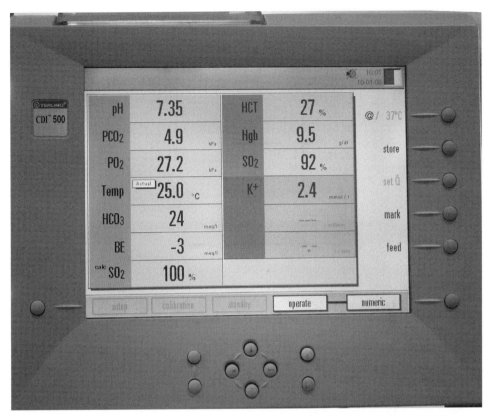

**Figure 1.14** Terumo CDI 500 in-line monitoring system, providing real-time blood gas, acid/base, Hb/HCT and electrolyte analysis.

The Terumo CDI 500 in-line blood gas analyzer is an optical fluorescence and reflectance based in-line system that continuously monitors 11 critical blood gas parameters with laboratory quality accuracy (see Figure 1.14). This level of sophistication and accuracy is, not surprisingly, expensive, and is reserved in many centers for particularly complex or prolonged cases – such as when gas analysis is changed from alpha-stat to pH-stat during the cooling or re-warming periods of procedures involving deep hypothermic circulatory arrest (DHCA).

There are more basic and commonly used forms of in-line monitoring available for use during CPB. Venous and arterial blood oxygen saturations can be continuously monitored during CPB using devices that rely on the absorbance or reflectance of infrared light signals. Although not always completely accurate, these devices are a valuable tool for observing and recording trends.

Non-invasive simultaneous arterial and venous saturation monitors are also available for use during CPB (see Figure 1.15). These have sensors that clip onto the outside of the venous and arterial tubing and continuously display venous and arterial saturations simultaneously on a computerized screen that is mounted on the frame of the CPB circuit. These tools all aid safe perfusion practice and are used in conjunction with laboratory blood gas analysis.

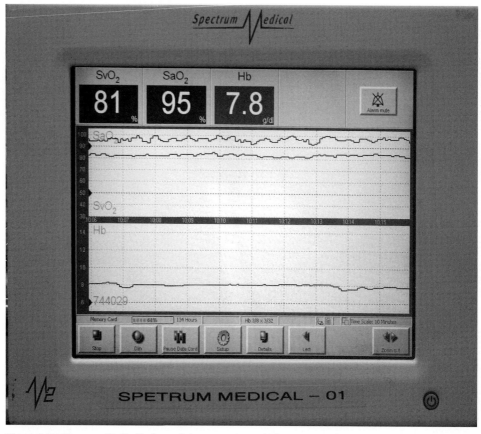

**Figure 1.15** Spectrum Medical in-line real-time saturation and Hb monitoring system.

## Alarms

Ideally all alarm systems are linked into the computer system of the CPB circuit and directly regulate or stop the pump flow when appropriate. The alarm systems used within the circuit aid the perfusionist in running a safe pump and are all vital components of the circuit. The alarms are engaged prior to initiating CPB and are not turned off, or over-ridden, until the patient has been weaned from CPB. The perfusionist, in an analogous fashion to a pilot, is the main safety device for the CPB circuit and constantly monitors all of the parameters associated with running the pump.

## Mini bypass system

There has been some recent interest in the development of miniature extracorporeal circuits (see Figure 1.16a). These are designed to reduce foreign surface area, priming volume (as little as 500 ml) and blood-air contact. This leads to decreased hemodilution, and thus reduced blood transfusion requirements, and may reduce the inflammatory response to CPB.

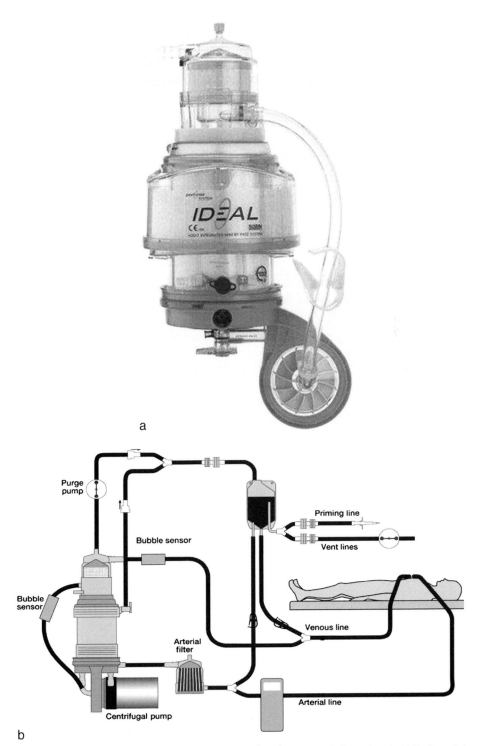

a

b

**Figure 1.16** (a) Mini bypass system. (b) Schematic drawing of mini bypass circuit. (Reproduced with kind permission from Sorin Group.)

Such circuits usually do not include a reservoir, heat exchanger and cardiotomy suction but increasingly incorporate arterial filters (see Figure 1.16b). Research and further development is ongoing, but early trials have been promising, some demonstrating a reduced release of vasoactive substances and a reduced activation of the coagulation cascade.

## Suggested Further Reading

- Anderson KS, Nygreen EL, Grong K, *et al.* Comparison of the centrifugal and roller pump in elective coronary bypass surgery: a prospective randomized study with a special emphasis upon platelet activation. *Scand Cardiovasc J* 2003; **37**: 356–62.

- Black S, Bolman RM III. C. Walton Lillehei and the birth of open heart surgery. *J Card Surg* 2006; **21**: 205–8.

- Driessen JJ, Dhaese H, Fransen G, *et al.* Pulsatile compared with non-pulsatile perfusion using a centrifugal pump for cardiopulmonary bypass during coronary artery bypass grafting: effects on systemic haemodynamics, oxygenation and inflammatory response parameters. *Perfusion* 1995; **10**: 3–12.

- Fried DW. Performance evaluation of blood-gas exchange devices. *Int Anesthesiol Clin* 1996; **34**: 47–60.

- Gibbon JH Jr. Development of the artificial heart and lung extracorporeal blood circuit. *JAMA* 1968; **206**: 1983–6.

- Kmiecik SA, Liu JL, Vaadia TS, *et al.* Quantative evaluation of hypothermia, hyperthermia and hemodilution on coagulation. *J Extra Corpor Technol* 2001; **33**: 100–5.

- Mejak BL, Stammers A, Rauch E, *et al.* A retrospective study on perfusion incidents and safety devices. *Perfusion* 2000; **15**: 51–61.

- Mulholland JW, Shelton JC, Luo XY. Blood flow and damage by the roller pumps during cardiopulmonary bypass. *J Fluid Struct* 2005; **20**: 129–40.

- Peek GJ, Thompson A, Killer HM, *et al.* Spallation performance of extracorporeal membrane oxygenation tubing. *Perfusion* 2000; **15**: 457–66.

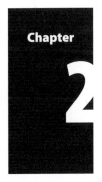

# Circuit setup and safety checks

Simon Colah and Steve Gray

Assembling the CPB circuit and checking the CPB machine for faults prior to clinical use is an essential part of the provision of extracorporeal perfusion. This chapter describes the procedure for "setting up" the CPB system and the safety checks that should be undertaken before embarking on a case.

Philip Kay and Christopher Munsch (2004) in "Techniques in Extracorporeal Circulation" state: "Cardiopulmonary bypass is a dynamic artificial environment conferring a shock state on the body with its own potential for severe morbidity and mortality." Vigilance is thus paramount to the conduct of cardiopulmonary bypass. Modern perfusion systems are designed to optimize safety. Technological advances have seen the incorporation of automatic alarms and fail-safe devices; however, the perfusionist's attention to detail and observance of prebypass checklists and protocols still underpins safe practice. Human error is a far greater cause of accidents than mechanical mishap.

Preparing the CPB circuit and machine, attention to the patient's clinical details and the surgical requirements for the procedure all form part of the process of safe provision of cardiopulmonary bypass. By necessity the preparation of the CPB machine and assembly of the disposable circuit components should be "ritualistic" following a routine dictated by institutional protocols.

## CPB machine preparation and circuit setup

CPB circuits are made up of a number of disposable items. Principally these are:

- the integrated membrane oxygenator/hardshell (or softshell) venous reservoir;
- cardioplegia set;
- arterial line filter; and
- custom tubing pack.

All components are rigorously checked. In particular, the disposable items are closely examined with regard to expiry date and integrity of the packaging.

There are many ways to set up a CPB circuit. Departmental preferences and specific patient requirements dictate the approach. A commonly used sequence for setting up and priming a standard CPB system is outlined in Appendix 2A, together with a synopsis of electronic safety devices in Appendix 2B, at the end of this chapter.

Securing the gas hoses to the gas source, checking that gas supplies of air and oxygen are functional and attaching the scavenging line initiates the process. The CPB machine console is then powered and temporarily disconnected to ascertain that the power failure alarm and backup battery unit are fully functional. Most operating rooms have an uninterruptible power supply (UPS), essentially a series of batteries linked to the hospital generator that powers the CPB machine, anesthetic machine, intravenous infusion pumps and other vital equipment

*Cardiopulmonary Bypass,* ed. S. Ghosh, F. Falter and D. J. Cook. Published by Cambridge University Press.
© Cambridge University Press 2009.

should there be a mains power failure. It must be ensured that the CPB machine is connected to a UPS.

The integrated oxygenator/venous reservoir is placed on its secure holder and orientated to allow full view of the reservoir. The oxygen/air delivery line and scavenging hose are attached to the appropriate ports on the base of the oxygenator. The sampling port manifold is positioned with taps secured. Tubing to the dedicated systemic, arterial flow pump is put into place and connected to the venous reservoir outlet and oxygenator inlet. The cardioplegia tubing is positioned, but not aligned at this stage, in the designated pump backplate. This expedites the priming of the cardioplegia circuit. The cardioplegia delivery system differs from the systemic flow pump or sucker pumps in that a pump which accommodates two segments of tubing with varying diameters within it may be used, so that blood and cardioplegia mixed in the desired ratio (usually 4 parts blood to 1 part cardioplegia) can be dispensed. Alternatively, two separate pumps may be used to independently deliver the blood and cardioplegia in a 4:1 ratio.

Roller pump heads are checked to ensure that they only rotate in one direction.

The arterio-venous loop (A-V loop), which when divided will be connected to the venous and arterial cannulae by the surgeon, is connected to the venous reservoir inlet and oxygenator outlet. The arterial line filter (with bypass link), pressure transducer and bubble detector are attached to the systemic flow tubing (see Fig. 1.1). The bubble detector is coupled to the CPB machine console so that if air is sensed in the arterial line an alarmed automatic pump cut out facility is activated. Likewise, the transduced pressure in the arterial line links to the CPB machine console, so that if the line pressure exceeds a set limit (usually 350 mmHg), through unintentional clamping or kinking, the pump will stop. This is preceded by slowing of the pump at a slightly lower pressure threshold (usually 300 mmHg). Suction and venting tubing (color coded for safety and ease of use) are then fixed into the various roller head assemblies. Two sets of water lines from the heater–cooler unit are attached to the oxygenator and blood cardioplegia heat exchange device. Water is circulated to ensure that there is no dangerous water leak.

The cardioplegia pressure transducer and purge lines are connected to the cardioplegia delivery device.

Just prior to priming, the arterial line filter is flushed with $CO_2$. Once flushed, the $CO_2$ is turned off and disconnected, the arterial line filter inlet and outlet and the cardioplegia delivery line are clamped off. The arterial line should also be clamped if there is a re-circulation shunt line distal to the arterial line filter. Some centers flush the whole circuit with $CO_2$ to displace air. This reduces the risk of gaseous emboli as carbon dioxide is nearly 30 times more soluble in blood than nitrogen.

One to two liters of prime fluid is added to the venous reservoir. The arterial pump is turned on at approximately 4–5 l/minute whilst the perfusionist observes prime filling the pump tubing, the oxygenator and any ancilliary lines. These must be closed or clamped after priming whilst fluid re-circulates via the arterial re-circulation line back into the venous reservoir. The arterial pressure dome is primed and secured to the transducer, the arterial line filter is retrogradely primed and its bypass line clamped. Flow through the A-V loop is established, left-recirculating and inspected for air bubbles, before clamping the re-circulation line. It is necessary to ensure that the cardioplegia circuit is primed and air free and that the pump occlusions have been adjusted, so that they are just "under-occlusive." The arterial and venous lines are then clamped and the prime allowed to re-circulate through the filter and purge lines.

There are two ways to check the roller heads for occlusion: either check each roller at the "6 o'clock" position or together at the "9.15" position, with the circuit pressurized at 250 mmHg and the arterial line clamped. Any rapid drop in pressure may indicate that connections are not secure or that an "occlusion" has been incorrectly set. Centrifugal pumps are non-occlusive and should be gravity filled to ensure good de-airing. Centrifugal consoles have integrated flow probes that are unidirectional. As they are afterload sensitive, pump speed must be set to produce forward flow before initiating bypass.

The inflow to the sucker pumps is clamped and the rollers are adjusted to avoid collapse of the tubing. The vent line should have a one-way pressure relief valve in-line to prevent inadvertent air entry into the heart and to prevent cavitation inside cardiac chambers.

Temperature probes are placed into the arterial, venous and cardiolegia ports and visualized on the LED display. The level sensor is placed at, or above, 400 ml and the bubble detector placed on the arterial line distal to the filter. All alarms, pressure ranges, timers and cardioplegia parameters can now be set in preparation for bypass.

## Design and use of a prebypass checklist

Experience from other high-risk industries, such as aviation or maritime, demonstrate that disasters are often associated with poor checking procedures. The format of the CPB checklist is either written or automated and best signed off by two perfusionists. Ideally, the primary perfusionist does the checking whilst the second perfusionist works through the list. The American Society of Extracorporeal Technology and the European Board of Cardiovascular Perfusion publish an excellent array of perfusion guidelines and checklists (see Figure 2.1). As expected the list is comprehensive yet targeted, covering all aspects from sterility to backup components.

## Safety concerns prior to, during and after CPB

Before embarking on a case the perfusionist should review the patient's notes. The most important details are:

- planned procedure and likelihood of additional procedures;
- allergies;
- significant comorbid conditions, such as diabetes or renal dysfunction; and
- metabolic or hematological abnormalities, such as anemia, thrombocytopenia or hyperkalemia.

The patient's blood group should be confirmed and the availability of bank blood checked.

Details of the patient's height and weight are essential to calculate:

- dose of heparin (usually 300 mg/kg) required for CPB;
- body surface area (BSA) in square meters, which is required to determine the "ideal" flow rate at normothermia (BSA × cardiac index) and so to select appropriately sized venous and arterial cannulae; and
- predicted HCT on initiation of CPB

Safety issues relating to the pre-, intra- and post-CPB periods are summarized in Tables 2.1, 2.2 and 2.3, respectively.

**Pre-bypass checklist**

☐ **Patient:** _____
☐ ID correct
☐ Chart reviewed

☐ **Sterility**
☐ Components: integrity and expiry date

☐ **Heart-lung machine**
☐ Power connected
☐ Start-up normal
☐ Back-up power

☐ **Heater-cooler**
☐ Start-up normal
☐ Water connections: flow verified
☐ Water temperature: _____ ° C/F

☐ **Gas supply**
☐ Gas lines connected
☐ Flow meter/blender in order
☐ Vaporizer shut off
☐ $CO_2$ flush

☐ **Pump**
☐ Roller heads not obstructed
☐ Flow meter: calibration & direction
☐ Tubing holders secure
☐ Occlusion set : _____ mmHg
      _____cmH$_2$0/min

☐ **Tubing**
☐ Pump tubing condition inspected
☐ Suckers functional and sucking
☐ One-way valves: direction correct
☐ Circuit shunts closed

☐ **ID:** _____

☐ **Monitoring**
☐ Temperature probes positioned
☐ Pressure transducers calibrated
☐ In/on-line sensors calibrated

☐ **Safety & alarms**
☐ Low-level alarm engaged
☐ Air detector engaged
☐ Pressure alarm limits set
☐ Temperature alarm limits set
☐ Cardiotomy reservoir vented

☐ **Oxygenator**
☐ Gas line attached
☐ Heat exchanger integrity inspected
☐ Scavenger attached

☐ **Debubbling**
☐ Tubing
☐ Oxygenator
☐ Cardioplegia
☐ Arterial filter/bubble trap

☐ **Accessories**
☐ Tubing clamps
☐ Hand cranks
☐ Backup circuit components

☐ **Anticoagulation**
☐ Heparin in: _____time
☐ Patient properly anticoagulated
☐ **Ready to start bypass**

☐ Signature: ........................................

**Figure 2.1.** Prebypass checklist. The European Board of Cardiovascular Perfusion (EBCP) promotes the use of prebypass checklists in the practice of clinical perfusion. The suggestions in this checklist are designed as the minimum requirements for cardiopulmonary bypass procedures and each institution should adapt this to suit its own requirements. The EBCP can accept no liability whatsoever for the adoption and practice of this suggested checklist. (Reproduced by kind permission of The European Board of Cardiovascular Perfusion: http://www.ebcp.org)

**Table 2.1.** Pre-CPB safety concerns

Heparin given, activated clotting time (ACT) >400 seconds

Arterial cannula correctly placed, pulsatile swing on an anaeroid pressure gauge connected to a side arm of the arterial line

Venous reservoir has a safe level of prime, additional fluid available to add, low level alarm activated

Oxygen analyzer monitoring gas supply to oxygenator on, alarm activated

Sweep rate appropriate for patient (usually 2–3 l, FiO$_2$ = 0.6)

Venous cannula relatively free of air

Shunt lines are clamped, apart from arterial filter purge line and drug administration manifold line

No clamps on the arterial or venous lines placed by surgical team

Alarm overrides deactivated

Vasopressors prescribed and available

**Table 2.2.** Safety concerns during CPB

| Concern | Common causes |
|---|---|
| Low level alarm on venous reservoir | Impaired venous return |
| | Tubing kinked |
| | Air lock |
| | Hemorrhage |
| | Misplaced venous canula |
| | Clotting within circuit |
| High-pressure alarm on arterial line | Clamping or kinking of line |
| | Manipulation of the aorta |
| | Clotting within circuit |
| | Aortic dissection |
| Bubble alarm | Air in line |
| | Sensor malfunction |
| Low mixed venous oxygen saturation | Erratic flow |
| | Considerable time spent with suboptimal flows |
| | Hemorrhage |
| | Depth of anesthesia lightening |
| | Shunt clamp inadvertently removed |
| | Excessive transfusion with non-blood products |
| Clotting | Inadequate heparinization |
| Poor blood gasses despite adequate sweep gas delivery and pump flow | Oxygenator failure |
| Electrical activity of the heart | Intervals between cardioplegia too long |
| | Too little cardioplegia delivered |
| | Aortic regurgitation |
| Hyperthermia | Overaggressive re-warming strategy |
| | Failure to maintain temperature gradient between heat exchanger and venous blood <10°C |

**Table 2.3.** Safety concerns on separating from CPB

| |
|---|
| Ventilation not established |
| Intracardiac vent still in place |
| Shunt lines open on CPB with the potential to exsanguinate the patient into circuit |
| Suction still in use during protamine administration |
| Inattention to level in venous reservoir whilst transfusing |
| Draining the venous line while cannula still positioned in the right atrium |
| Dismantling the CPB circuit before hemodynamic stability has been achieved |

**Table 2.4.** Key factors contributing to a safer perfusion service

| |
|---|
| Accreditation of training programs |
| Certification and re-certification of perfusionists |
| Conferences, yearly appraisals, departmental quality assurance meetings |
| Reporting of adverse occurrences |
| Quality in-house training |
| Electronic data acquisition with associated audit facilities |
| Departmental protocols, especially outlining procedures in abnormal and emergency situations |
| Manufacturer product alerts acted on |
| Equipment maintenance records and quality assurance logs kept |

## Conclusion

Surveys by Jenkins *et al.* (1997) and Mejak *et al.* (2000) report the number of pump-related incidents to be 1:140 and the likelihood of permanent injury or death of the patient after such an incident to be 1:1350. A multitude of healthcare organizations, not least the Institute of Medicine (IOM), have called for a 90% reduction in preventable patient injuries.

Since the introduction of CPB in the early 1950s the focus on safety has evolved and improved. Today, the quality of components is excellent. CPB machines incorporate in-built alarms with auto-regulatory feedback systems, together with real-time data acquisition. Yet surveys confirm the mishap rate is slow to fall. Accredited training, scrupulous attention to detail and use of checklists and protocols will hopefully continue to improve safety. The key factors contributing to a safer perfusion service are summarized in Table 2.4.

# Appendix 2A: Procedure for setting up and priming a standard heart–lung bypass system

(Adapted, with permission, from London Perfusion Science Protocols.)

## 2A.1: The heart–lung machine and accessories

### 2A1.1: Connection checks

(a)   All cables, plugs and sockets are checked
(b)   All cables should be laid neatly, so that they are not likely to be damaged and where they are least likely to cause accidents
(c)   All parts of the apparatus, including heater/chiller and pump light (if it is to be used) are checked for power
(d)   Gas lines are fitted to the wall outlets and connections, hoses, mixers and flow meters are checked for leaks
(e)   Gas flow to the oxygenator is checked

### 2A1.2: Pump head checks

Each pump head is checked:

(a)   For power

(b)     The rollers and guides are moving
(c)     The pump heads are free from foreign bodies
(d)     The pump heads are set to rotate in the correct direction
(e)     The flow/rpm settings on the console are accurately calibrated
(f)     For winding handles
(g)     That the tubing inserts are of the correct size for the tubing to be used

## 2A1.3: Checks that other electrical safety devices are in working order

(a)     Battery backup (UPS) is charged
(b)     Pressure transducers
(c)     Level detectors
(d)     Bubble detectors

# 2A.2: The setup of disposable heart–lung equipment

## 2A2.1: The oxygenator

(a)     Remove packaging and check its integrity and sterility
(b)     The oxygenator is examined for obvious faults and debris
(c)     The oxygenator is placed securely into its holder
(d)     Any gas outflow cap is removed
(e)     The gas connection is made
(f)     Remove any venting cap on the reservoir
(g)     The $CO_2$ flush is initiated until priming
(h)     The water connections to the heater/chiller are now made, the heat exchanger and all connections are checked for leaks with the water running at 37°C

## 2A2.2: The circuitry

(a)     Remove packaging and check its integrity and sterility
(b)     The circuitry is checked for faults (cracked connectors, kinked tubing, etc.)
(c)     Check the silicone pump boot and place so it is lying correctly in order to prevent wear or damage from the tube guides or rollers
(d)     Check that the pump boot tube is securely held at both the outlet and the inlet. Rotate the pump to check the tubing is correctly seated
(e)     Do the same with sucker tubing, checking direction of flow
(f)     With attention to sterile technique, connect the pump lines to the oxygenator, ensure they have been connected in the correct direction and not crossed over
(g)     The lines should be sufficiently long so that they may be moved to the neighboring pump head if necessary
(h)     Any cuts to tubing should be made cleanly and perpendicular to the length of the tubing, using a sterile blade
(i)     The outflow line should now be connected to the outflow port of the oxygenator
(j)     The re-circulating lines should now be similarly connected as required by manufacturer's specifications
(k)     All pressure connections can be made secure using nylon ties

## 2A2.3: The cardiotomy reservoir if required

(a)     The reservoir can be used for any surgery where intracardiac clot is suspected, where it is anticipated that large quantities of blood will be used or where the use of auto transfusion is anticipated

(b)     The reservoir and its packaging is checked as above and inserted into the appropriate holder

(c)     Remove any venting cap and using the 3/8″ cardiotomy return, connect the cardiotomy to the oxygenator, ensuring that this return line cannot be kinked or obstructed

(d)     Connect the sucker lines and recirculation lines to the cardiotomy reservoir

## 2A2.4: The cardioplegia system if required

(a)     Remove packaging and check its integrity and sterility

(b)     The circuitry is checked for faults (cracked connections, kinked tubing, etc.)

(c)     Assemble circuit according to manufacturer's instructions

(d)     Ensure all connections (oxygenator, recirculation lines, etc.) are secure and correct

(e)     Water lines are connected to the cardioplegia administration set heat exchanger. Water is circulated to ensure that it is free from leaks

## 2A2.5: The centrifugal pump if required

(a)     Remove packaging and check its integrity and sterility

(b)     The relevant flow and drive connectors should be connected to the console

(c)     The battery charger should be examined to determine whether or not there is sufficient battery backup

(d)     The perfusionist should check that the relevant hand-crank mechanism is available in case of power failure

(e)     The drive motor heads must be examined for dirt, as this may impair the function of the device, including the possibility of disengagement

## 2A2.6: Arterial line filters if required

(a)     Check the filter for sterility, any damage or debris

(b)     If the filter is to be cut into the arterial line this should be carried out using the appropriate sterile technique

(c)     Ensure the filter holder is positioned to prevent the stretching or kinking of lines

(d)     Position the filter securely in the holder

An air bubble trap would be primed in a similar fashion.

## 2A2.7: Cell saver if required

(a)     Remove outer packaging and check its integrity and sterility

(b)     Open the collection reservoir portion of the set and secure firmly in holder

(c)     Connect the vacuum source to the reservoir

(d)     The washing portion of the set should only be opened when either enough blood has been collected to salvage or the perfusionist is confident that enough blood will be collected to salvage

(e) The washing portion of the set should be assembled neatly
(f) All ports and connections should be checked, closed and tightened where necessary

## 2A2.8: Prebypass filters if used

If the circuit contains a prebypass filter there are a number of points the perfusionist must remember:

- The prebypass filter should be removed before priming the circuit with blood
- The prebypass filter should be removed if the low pressure suction is required before the lines have been divided

A ½" × 3/8" connector should be readily available to replace the prebypass filter if necessary.

# 2A.3: In-line blood chemistry/gas analyzer (e.g., CDI 500) setup and calibration

## 2A3.1: Setup of CDI 500 arterial sensor shunt

(a) Turn off monitor and after the monitor has self-tested select the required configuration of the sensor shunt
(b) Select calibration
(c) Verify the K* calibration value on the sensor packaging
(d) Check that the calibrator's cable is connected to the monitor
(e) Remove blue cap from the base of the sensor shunt and attach to one of the calibrator's ports
(f) Loosen the blue cap on the top of the sensor shunt
(g) Initiate calibration by pressing √ twice on the monitor
(h) Calibration lasts 10 minutes
(i) After calibration tighten large luer cap and remove gas filter

## 2A3.2: Setup of CDI 500 Venous Line Sensor

(a) Remove venous sensor from packaging and cut into venous line
(b) After the monitor has been switched on and has self-tested the venous probe can be connected to the venous sensor

# 2A.4: Priming the system

The perfusionist should ensure, if possible, that the following patient details are available from the anesthetic and surgical staff, to provide a basis on which to decide the priming strategy:

- Height and weight
- Renal status
- Hb/HCT
- Heart size
- Fluid status

## 2A4.1: Standard prime

(a)  1 l Hartmann's solution is checked

(b)  Preservative-free heparin should be injected into the liter bag of Hartmann's solution (dose per liter of prime as per institutional protocol) and labeled

(c)  The Hartmann's solution is run into the system via a giving set or rapid prime line. It is important that this heparinized prime runs through the length of the circuit (i.e., all filters are exposed to this heparinized prime). The prime is delivered via a cardiotomy port (if a cardiotomy is in use)

(d)  The reservoir should be inspected for obvious bubbles and tapped to remove them

(e)  Sufficient prime should be added to the system to maintain a dynamic priming volume

(f)  It is most important at this stage that the oxygenator manufacturer's instructions are carefully adhered to

(g)  Turn off the $CO_2$ flush

(h)  A gravity feed prime is undertaken, with de-bubbling taking place in a logical fashion, beginning with the oxygenator reservoir and progressing to the arterial line and so on

(i)  The "sash" should be clamped off, the arterial pump switched on and the prime re-circulated

(j)  The pressure line may now be connected, via an air-free isolator to the line pressure gauge and pressure transducer

(k)  The re-circulation lines are securely clamped, and the "sash" primed

(l)  It is important to remember that air is easily dragged across the membrane of hollow fiber oxygenators, so the following precautions should be taken to avoid this:

  • the venous line should be partially occluded so as to offer a resistance, and therefore maintain a positive pressure as the prime is re-circulating
  • the pump should be switched off slowly to avoid the momentum effect (see below)

(m)  When the circuit appears to be clear of bubbles, the re-circulation rate should now be increased to around 5 l/minute, to remove any bubbles from within the oxygenator membrane with the venous line partially clamped maintaining a post-membrane pressure of around 80 mmHg. Before the "sash" is divided, a final check must be made by both perfusionist and surgeon for the presence of bubbles. Before stopping the re-circulation, the pump should be turned down slowly, reducing the chances of the inertia effect of a sudden reduction in flow that would cause air to be dragged across the membrane

## 2A4.2: Priming cardioplegia if required

(a)  The type, temperature and concentration of blood cardioplegia should be determined from the surgeon in advance. This information should be held in the hospital's database (e.g., proportion 4:1, 2:1, etc., the need for any "hot shots," etc.)

(b)  Bags of Ringer's solution should be carefully prepared. The vials of cardioplegia should be carefully checked before injection. The bags must be labeled clearly as soon as this has been done

(c) The cardioplegia circuit is primed with Hartmann's solution or Ringer's solution, checking that all air has been purged

(d) During priming, care must be taken that the main prime does not become contaminated with cardioplegia

(e) The cardioplegia pump boots are placed in the raceway and appropriately sized collets fitted (if applicable), or a check is made to ensure that the ratio is correctly programed into the pump console

(f) The occlusion of the pump is then set as with the arterial pump (see later)

## 2A4.3: Priming the arterial line filter if required

(a) Place clamps either side of the arterial filter before the oxygenator is gravity primed

(b) Once the circuit is primed, stop the pump, slowly release lower clamp and allow prime to flow retrogradely through the filter via the bypass line, expelling air through the purge line. The retrograde flow is provided by the prime in the "sash"

(c) Release the top clamp, start the pump

(d) Invert the filter and de-air as normal

(e) Clamp the arterial filter bypass loop

## 2A4.4: Priming centrifugal pump if required

Centrifugal pumps differ from roller pumps in several important respects:

• They are non-occlusive devices
• They are constant energy devices

(a) A length of 3/8″ PVC tubing is connected to the outlet of the venous reservoir and clamped. A length of 3/8″ PVC tubing is also connected to the oxygenator inlet port

(b) The outlet of the membrane compartment is connected to the circuit as with a roller pump

(c) If a "BioPump" bi-directional flow probe is required it should be inserted into the arterial line, at least 6″ away from the nearest connector

(d) The oxygenator venous reservoir is primed with heparinized Hartmann's solution, as described in the routine procedure

(e) The centrifugal pump is cut in as required ensuring sterile technique using a sterile blade

(f) The clamp on the inlet tube is then slowly released, allowing the prime to slowly fill the head. The outlet port of the head (which is tangential to the body of the head) is held uppermost. The head is thus filled with the priming solution, and as much air as possible is purged

(g) The oxygenator is gravity primed as above

(h) The head should again be examined for bubbles and if found should be manipulated out of the inlet port back into the venous reservoir

(i) When the outlet of the centrifugal head is clamped any air will collect at the center of the casing (low mass). If the pump is then switched off the collected air will travel vertically into the inlet tube. As before, this air can be manipulated back into the venous reservoir

## 2A4.5: Calibrating the flow probes

With the circuit fully primed:

(a)   The motor drive is switched off
(b)   Clamps are positioned some 6″ on either side of the probe
(c)   Calibrate the flow probe as directed by manufacturer's instructions

## 2A.5: Setting occlusions

### 2A5.1: Occlusion of the arterial pump if a roller pump is used:

(a)   Clamp the arterial line and any re-circulating lines and close the sampling ports
(b)   The pump is carefully turned until the pressure on the gauge is around 300 mmHg and the rate of fall of pressure can be observed
(c)   Tighten the occlusion until there is no fall of pressure in this high-pressure range (this ensures that there are no other leaks in the circuit and that all clamps are competent)
(d)   Adjust the occlusion until the fall off of pressure over the lower 260–280 mmHg range takes approximately 10 seconds
(e)   Both rollers must be treated individually. Should the occlusion between rollers be obviously unequal, the pump should be changed

### 2A5.2: Occlusion of the suction pumps

(a)   A clamp is placed on the negative side of the sucker boot and the pump is turned until the boot collapses with the vacuum created
(b)   The occlusion should now be "backed off" until the vacuum is cleared
(c)   The occlusion setting is then again increased, until the vacuum is just drawn and held
(d)   In order to check the direction of rotation of the sucker/vent roller pumps, a small quantity of heparinized saline or other appropriate fluid should be used by the scrub nurse to check the suction

## Appendix 2B: Electronic safety devices

(Adapted, with permission, from London Perfusion Science Protocols.)

## 2B.1: Level sensors

• The level sensor should be positioned at around the 400 ml mark on the reservoir
• If the option is available, level sensors should be set to slow the pump down before stopping it
• Level sensors should not be overridden unless it is absolutely necessary

## 2B.2: Bubble detectors

• Perfusionists must use a gas bubble detector placed in the circuit: it is usual practice to have the bubble detector on the arterial outlet of the circuit

## 2B.3: Pressure alarms

- Most modern heart-lung machines have integrated electronic alarms for limits of pressure during a case
- These limits should be checked and correctly set to appropriate parameters before each case

## 2B.4: Temperature alarms

- Most modern heart-lung machines have integrated electronic alarms for limits of temperature during a case
- Arterial blood, venous blood and cardioplegia temperature alarms should be checked and correctly set to appropriate parameters before each case
- Where available the water temperature alarm limits should also be checked and set

## 2B.5: Gas alarms

- Most modern gas blenders have alarms for gas failure
- These alarms can be checked when the gas lines are connected to the hospital gas supply
- Connecting the lines then disconnecting them individually should trigger the alarm

## 2B.6: Electrical failure alarm

- Most modern heart-lung machines have an integrated alarm that sounds when the mains power supply fails and UPS is activated. If this occurs, all unnecessary equipment should be turned off to conserve the battery.

## Suggested Further Reading

- American Society of Extra-Corporeal Technology, Herndon, VA. www.amsect.org

- Gravlee GP, Davis RF, Stammers AH, Ungerleider RM. *Cardiopulmonary Bypass Principles and Practice.* 3rd edition, 2008, Lippincott Williams & Wilkins.

- Jenkins OF, Morris R, Simpson JM. Australian perfusion incident survey. *Perfusion* 1997; **12**: 279–288.

- Kay PH, Munsch CM. *Techniques in Extracorporeal Circulation.* 4th edition, 2004. London: Arnold.

- Mejak BL, Stammers A, Rauch E, *et al.* A retrospective study on perfusion incidents and safety devices. *Perfusion* 2000; **15**: 51–61.

- Recommendations for Standards of Monitoring during Cardiopulmonary Bypass. Published by the: Society of Clinical Perfusion Scientists of Great Britain & Ireland, Association of Cardiothoracic Anaesthetists, Society of Cardiothoracic Surgeons in Great Britain & Ireland. July 2007.

- Wheeldon DR. Safety during cardiopulmonary bypass. *London: Franklin Scientific Projects*, 1986; **7**: 57–65.

# Chapter 3

# Priming solutions for cardiopulmonary bypass circuits

George Hallward and Roger Hall

The cardiopulmonary bypass (CPB) circuit must be primed with a fluid solution, so that adequate flow rates can be rapidly achieved on initiation of CPB without risk of air embolism. The optimum composition of the CPB priming solution is still a matter for debate. Currently used "primes" have evolved from historical concepts of using a solution with similar electrolyte content and osmolarity to the intravascular and interstitial compartments, providing a fluid that when mixed with blood is capable of maintaining oxygen delivery, carbon dioxide removal and physiological homeostasis.

## Prime volume

The volume of prime required is either based on a standard empirically derived volume greater than a minimum safe priming volume, or may be guided by the patient's weight or body surface area. In practice, the minimum volume required is that which fills both venous and arterial limbs of the circuit and maintains an adequate reserve volume in the venous reservoir to ensure that air is not entrained into the arterial side of the circuit during initiation of CPB. This volume is determined by both the caliber and length of tubing connecting the patient to the CPB machine and by the design, and therefore capacity, of the venous reservoir and oxygenator. Reduction of the prime volume may thus be achieved by modification of the circuit.

The initial hematocrit (HCT) achieved after initiation of CPB is determined by the volume of the prime in relation to the patient's pre-CPB HCT. In adults, priming volumes are commonly in the range of 1400–1800 ml, typically representing 30–35% of the patient's blood volume. In children, especially infants and neonates, even the minimum priming volume is often far greater than their blood volume, making the use of non-blood-containing primes impossible.

## Acceptable hemodilution

Initiation of CPB inevitably leads to hemodilution by the priming fluid. Some degree of hemodilution is beneficial as blood viscosity is reduced, improving microcirculatory flow. Most centers aim for an HCT of less than 30% during CPB; however, there is no consensus regarding optimal HCT. HCT is the main determinant of the oxygen-carrying capacity of blood. Theoretically, minimum acceptable HCT should meet the oxygen delivery ($DO_2$) required to match systemic $O_2$ consumption ($VO_2$). However, $DO_2$ is influenced by pump flow rate and systemic temperature and $VO_2$ also alters proportionately with temperature. There is thus wide variation in practice with regard to the minimum, safe, acceptable HCT. Values as low as 14% have been advocated by some, whilst others have suggested using venous oxygen saturation ($S_vO_2$) rather than a specific HCT value as transfusion trigger. Experience with

*Cardiopulmonary Bypass*, ed. S. Ghosh, F. Falter and D. J. Cook. Published by Cambridge University Press.

Jehovah's Witness patients who refuse blood transfusions show that cardiac surgery and CPB with low HCTs is not only possible, but is also relatively safe.

Factors affecting the HCT during CPB include:

- patient size;
- preoperative hemoglobin concentration/HCT;
- pre-CPB blood loss;
- pre-CPB fluid administration;
- CPB prime volume; and
- urine output.

One method of reducing the degree of hemodilution, without using "Bank" blood, is to use autologous blood to partially prime the CPB circuit. This method replaces part of the CPB prime volume with the patient's own blood thus reducing the degree of hemodilution. Autologous priming can be achieved by either antegrade or retrograde routes. Antegrade priming utilizes partial filling of the venous reservoir with the patient's own blood from the venous limb of the CPB circuit on initiation of CPB, but before institution of CPB flow through the oxygenator and arterial limb of the circuit. Retrograde priming utilizes retrograde filling of the venous reservoir via the arterial limb of the CPB circuit, just prior to the initiation of CPB, displacing the crystalloid prime volume in the arterial line tubing, filter and oxygenator and so partially filling the reservoir with the patient's blood. Both methods reduce the volume of crystalloid in the prime by replacing it with 400–500 ml of the patient's blood. Safe autologous priming relies on good teamwork between perfusionist, anesthetist and surgeon to select appropriate patients and to ensure hemodynamic stability, usually with the help of vasopressors, during the period of partial exsanguination of the patient.

In general, acceptance of a degree of hemodilution during CPB, the use of autologous priming, collection and processing of shed mediastinal blood and the return of residual pump blood at the end of CPB can all lead to a decrease in allogenic blood transfusions with their consequent risks and uncertain risk/benefit profile.

## Priming solutions

There are many different recipes for priming solutions using crystalloid, colloid or blood as primary constituents. Historically, blood was used to prime the CPB circuit in an attempt to preserve a high hematocrit; early in the evolution of CPB this was thought to be an important determinant for successful outcome. It later became clear, however, that use of allogenic blood in the prime may have worsened, rather than improved, outcomes. In 1962, Cooley and coworkers showed improved outcome by adding 5% dextrose to the prime instead of just blood. Five percent dextrose later fell out of favor for two reasons: firstly, the realization that metabolism of glucose leads to a hypotonic solution; and secondly, fears about hyperglycemia worsening neurological outcome. In part, accumulation of knowledge about the deleterious effects of blood primes and acceptance that a lower hematocrit is compatible with good outcomes has led to acceptance of crystalloids as priming solutions. The introduction of hypothermic bypass in the 1960s, the inability of blood banks to support cardiac surgery with large amounts of whole blood and the prevalence of blood-borne infections were also important in the shift to "clear" primes. In general, an ideal priming solution should have the same tonicity, electrolyte composition and pH as that of plasma. Of these ideal properties the most important is that of "tonicity," in order to avoid red cell lysis and the fluid shifts from the extracellular to the intracellular compartment that occur with hypotonic solutions. Fluid shifts may occur in any organ or tissue, but the organs most vulnerable to fluid accumulation are the brain and lungs. Intracellular fluid gain causes cerebral or pulmonary edema and impairs organ function. It is important to appreciate that fluids which are nominally isotonic but which have glucose as a major constituent, e.g., 5% dextrose or dextrose/saline, become very hypotonic when the glucose is metabolized. For this reason, glucose-containing solutions should not be a major constituent of a prime and only those fluids with a near physiological sodium concentration should be used.

Suitable solutions used include lactated Ringer's (Hartmann's), Ringer's, normal saline, Plasma-Lyte and Normosol (see Tables 3.1 and 3.2). All of these solutions have similar sodium concentrations (130–150 mmol/l) and may contain physiological concentrations of potassium (Hartmann's, Plasma-Lyte). There are some differences in anion composition, but all have chloride as a major anionic constituent, the balance in Hartmann's or Plasma-Lyte being made up with lactate or acetate, respectively. Both lactate and acetate are ultimately metabolized to bicarbonate in the liver, thus producing a near ideal physiological solution. Hartmann's solution is the most commonly used crystalloid in priming fluids in the UK, although there is variation in practice amongst different units. Normosol-A and Plasma-Lyte are balanced solutions more commonly used in the USA.

The priming solution has been implicated as one of the potential causes of the disturbance of pH associated with development of metabolic acidosis on initiation of CPB. This acidosis is probably caused by hyperchloremia and is more likely to occur with normal saline, which has a higher chloride load than the more "physiological" solutions. Other possible reasons for this include an increase in unmeasured anions such as acetate and gluconate. This metabolic

**Table 3.1.** Composition of commonly used priming fluids

| | Na⁺ | K⁺ | Cl⁻ | Ca²⁺ | Mg²⁺ | HCO₃⁻ | pH | Other | mosmol/l |
|---|---|---|---|---|---|---|---|---|---|
| Dextrose 5% | 0 | 0 | 0 | 0 | 0 | 0 | 4.2 | Glucose 50 g/l | 279 |
| Saline 0.9% | 154 | 0 | 154 | 0 | 0 | 0 | 5.0 | – | 308 |
| Hartmann's | 131 | 5.0 | 111 | 2.0 | 0 | 29 (lactate) | 6.5 | – | 280 |
| Plasmalyte A | 140 | 5.0 | 98 | 0 | 3 | 27 (acetate) | 7.4 | – | 294 |
| | | | | | | 29 (gluconate) | | | |
| Normasol R | 140 | 5.0 | 98 | 0 | 3 | 27 (acetate) | 7.4 | – | 294 |
| | | | | | | 29 (gluconate) | | | |
| Bicarbonate 1.26% | 150 | 0 | 0 | 0 | 0 | 150 | 7.0 | – | 300 |
| Gelofusine | 154 | 0.4 | 120 | 0.4 | 0 | 0 | 7.1–7.7 | Gelatine 40 g/l | 274 |
| Starch | 154 | 0 | 154 | 0 | 0 | 0 | 4.5–5.5 | Starch | 308 |
| Human Albumin 4.5 | 100–160 | <2 | 100–160 | 0 | 0 | <0.1 citrate | 7.1 | Albumin 40–50 g/l | 300 |

**Table 3.2.** Commonly used additives

| | |
|---|---|
| Heparin | 1000–2500 U/l of prime to ensure adequate anticoagulation |
| Bicarbonate | 25 mmol/l of prime as buffer when unbalanced priming solutions are used |
| Mannitol | Osmotic diuretic and free radical scavenger |
| Calcium | Needed if citrated blood is added to the prime to prevent chelation of calcium |
| Steroids | To attenuate systemic inflammatory response to CPB (evidence weak) |

acidosis is a benign phenomenon and probably accounts for much of the base deficit observed while on bypass.

Colloid solutions, including 4.5% albumin, gelatins, e.g., gelofusine, dextrans and starches, e.g., hydroxyethyl starch, have been advocated for use in the CPB prime on account of their potential to counteract the decrease in colloid oncotic pressure associated with hemodilution of albumin and other circulating plasma proteins during CPB. This reduction in colloid oncotic pressure causes movement of water out of the intravascular space and into the interstitial and intracellular spaces, contributing to postoperative edema and subsequent organ dysfunction. Thus, using colloids, with their high molecular weight, to maintain oncotic pressure and therefore reduce fluid shifts seems an attractive strategy. The drawback to this hypothesis is that whilst, in theory, colloid solutions ought to remain in the intravascular space, in practice the "tight junctions," which render the endothelial lining impermeable to large molecules, become more permeable on activation of the systemic inflammatory response associated with CPB. This may paradoxically increase the amount of extravasated fluid, as the high-molecular-weight constituents of colloid solutions become trapped in the interstitial fluid, potentially adding to edema by drawing more free fluid into the interstitium. Furthermore, some of the constituents of colloids have undesirable properties: dextrans interfere with coagulation, starches may remain in the body for years, with unknown long-term consequences and albumin solutions are in scarce supply and pose infection hazards. Cost and availability are also an issue with colloid solutions.

The use of colloid-based primes has not been shown to significantly influence clinical outcomes such as the duration of ventilatory support and length of intensive care unit (ICU) or hospital stay. None of the types of colloids has been shown to have significant advantages over another. Albumin may have a beneficial effect as a constituent of the prime: it is thought to coat the extracorporeal circuit, making it appear less "foreign" to the body's immune mechanisms and so to ameliorate the inflammatory response.

The lack of measurable benefit, potential risks and the significant cost penalty incurred in comparison to crystalloid fluids have resulted in colloids no longer being widely used as a priming fluid in adult CPB.

The use of mannitol as a colloidal fluid added to the CPB prime is perhaps the one exception to the above discussion. Mannitol is a common constituent of primes, but the indication for its use is for its properties as a potent osmotic diuretic, rather than to simply raise the oncotic pressure of the prime. Maintenance of urine output both during CPB and in the immediate postoperative period is desirable to enhance elimination from the body of the fluid load presented by prebypass iv fluids, the priming fluid volume and cardioplegia solution. It has also been postulated that mannitol may help to preserve renal function and reduce the incidence of post-CPB renal dysfunction, although the evidence for this is extremely weak. In addition, mannitol is a free radical scavenger and it is appealing to think that the free radicals produced during periods of hypoperfusion, ischemia and reperfusion might be "mopped up" during bypass, thus reducing end-organ damage. However, this concept remains unproven in any clinically relevant way.

## Experimental oxygen-carrying solutions

The idea of using oxygen-carrying solutions as blood substitutes may be an attractive means of maintaining oxygen delivery. They would address the expense, limited supply and disease transmission associated with blood transfusion. Both hemoglobin-based substitutes and per-fluorocarbons have been researched in the context of use in the CPB priming fluid, but none have yet proven to be both safe and efficacious as alternatives for oxygen carriage. Despite several decades of research no molecule seems close to being marketed as a viable alternative to red cells in the clinical arena and it remains to be seen whether there is any future for the use of these oxygen-carrying solutions during CPB.

## Suggested Further Reading

- Bunn F, Alderson P, Hawkins V. Colloid solutions for fluid resuscitation. *Cochrane Database Syst Rev* 2003; Art No CD001319(1):1–40.

- Cooley DA, Beall AC, Grondin P. Open heart operations with disposable oxygenators, 5% dextrose prime, and normothermia. *Surgery* 1962; **52**:713–19.

- Fang WC, Helm RE, Krieger KH, *et al.* Impact of minimum haematocrit during cardiopulmonary bypass on mortality in patients undergoing coronary artery surgery. *Circulation* 1997; **96**(suppl II): II-194–99.

- Harris EA, Seelye ER, Barratt-Boyes BG. Respiratory and acid-base changes during CPB in man. *Br J Anaesth* 1970; **42** : 912–21.

- Hoeft A, Korb H, Mehlhorn U, *et al.* Priming of cardiopulmonary bypass with human albumin or ringer lactate: effect on colloid osmotic pressure and extravascular lung water. *Br J Anaesth* 1991; **66**:73–80.

- Klein HG, Spahn DR, Carson JL. Red blood cell transfusion in clinical practice. *Lancet* 2007; **370**(9585):,415–26.

- Lilley A. The selection of priming fluids for cardiopulmonary bypass in the UK and Ireland. *Perfusion* 2002; **17**:315–319.

- Liskaser FJ, Bellomo R, Hayhoe M, *et al.* Role of pump prime in etiology and pathogenesis of cardiopulmonary bypass – associated acidosis. *Anesthesiology* 2000; **93** : 1170–3.

- Marelli D, Paul A, Samson R, *et al.* Does the addition of albumin to the prime solution in cardiopulmonary bypass affect outcome? A prospective randomized study. *J Thorac Cardiovasc Surg* 1989; **98**(5 Pt1): 751–6.

- Paone G, Silverman N. The paradox of on bypass transfusion thresholds in blood conservation. *Circulation* 1997; **96**(suppl II): II-205–8.

- Rawn JD. Blood transfusion in cardiac surgery: a silent epidemic revisited. *Circulation* 2007; **116**(22): 2523–4.

- Riegger L, Voepel-Lewis T, Kulik T, *et al.* Albumin versus crystalloid prime solution for cardiopulmonary bypass in young children. *Crit Care Med* 2002; **30**(12): 2649–54.

- Rosengart TK, DeBois WJ, Helm RE. Retrograde autologous priming (RAP) for cardiopulmonary bypass: a safe and effective means of decreasing hemodilution and transfusion requirements. *J Thorac Cardiovasc Surg* 1998; **115**(2): 426–38.

- Rosengart TK, Helm RE, DeBois WJ. Open heart operations without transfusion using a multimodality blood conservation strategy in 50 Jehovah's Witness patients: implications for a "bloodless" surgical technique. *J Am Coll Surg* 1997; **184**: 618–29.

- Russell JA, Navickis RJ, Wilkes MM. Albumin versus crystalloid for pump priming in cardiac surgery: a meta-analysis of controlled trials. *J Cardiothorac Vasc Anesth* 2004; **18**(4): 429–37.

- Serious Hazards of Transfusion, http://www.shotuk.org.

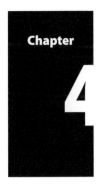

# Chapter 4

# Anticoagulation, coagulopathies, blood transfusion and conservation

Liza Enriquez and Linda Shore-Lesserson

Anticoagulation is required for any form of extracorporeal circulation to prevent activation of the coagulation system by contact between blood and artificial, non-biological surfaces.

Cardiopulmonary bypass circuits comprise of a large surface area of mainly plastic material, which if left to come into contact with blood without appropriate anticoagulation, would result in formation of clots within the circuit in a matter of minutes. In order to safely conduct CPB for the duration required for surgical procedures, or to maintain patients on extracorporeal support, anticoagulation must be adequate to prevent the development of even "minor" clots. Inadequate anticoagulation can in its most serious form lead to death and in lesser forms lead to impairment of organ function, usually manifest as neurological or renal dysfunction. Furthermore, any clots within the CPB system can trigger the development of disseminated intravascular coagulation (DIC), which results in the rapid consumption of clotting factors and failure of the body's coagulation system.

Heparin is the most commonly used anticoagulant in the context of CPB. This chapter describes the coagulation pathway, the pharmacology of heparin, monitoring of anticoagulation status, problems associated with heparin usage, alternatives to heparin, the reversal of anticoagulation following termination of CPB and the prevention and management of bleeding.

## The coagulation cascade

Coagulation occurs by interaction of a series of proteins that are activated and propagated by a variety of stimuli, including contact with foreign surfaces, contact with receptors on the surfaces of platelets and by factors produced by the systemic inflammatory response, all of which are pertinent in the context of CPB.

Most of the proteins required for the cascade are produced by the liver as inactive precursors which are then modified into clotting factors. The implication of the term "cascade" is that a small stimulus results in a reaction which may be amplified to produce a significant clot.

There are two routes for activation of the coagulation system. The intrinsic pathway is activated by contact with collagen from damaged blood vessels or any negatively charged surface. Platelet activation is normally involved. The extrinsic pathway is activated by contact with tissue factor from the surface of extravascular cells. Both routes end in a final common pathway – the proteolytic activation of thrombin and the cleaving of fibrinogen to form a fibrin clot. The intrinsic pathway is the predominant route, with the extrinsic pathway acting synergistically (see Figure 4.1).

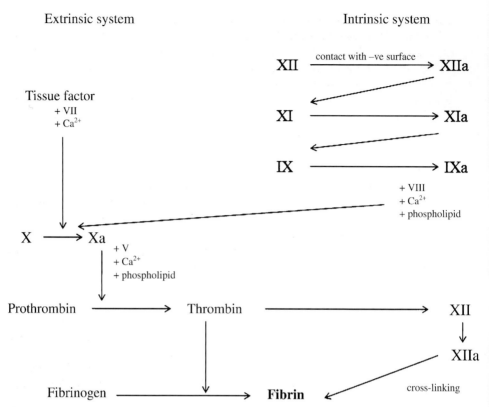

**Figure 4.1.** Overview of extrinsic and intrinsic clotting pathways.

# Pharmacological strategies for anticoagulation during CPB

## Heparin

Unfractionated heparin (UFH) remains the standard anticoagulant for CBP for several reasons. It is relatively safe, easy to use, has a fast onset of action and is measurable, titratable and reversible. It is also cost-effective.

### Structure

Native heparin is a polymer with a molecular weight ranging from 3 to 40 kDa, although the average molecular weight of most commercial heparin preparations is in the range of 12–15 kDa. Heparin is a member of the glycosaminoglycan family of carbohydrates (which includes the closely related molecule heparan sulfate) and consists of a variably sulfated repeating disaccharide unit that is negatively charged at physiological pH. Heparin is normally released by mast cells and basophils in the body and is commercially derived from bovine lung or porcine intestinal mucosa.

### Mechanism of anticoagulant action

Heparin contains a specific pentasaccharide sulfation sequence that binds to the enzyme inhibitor antithrombin III (AT-III) causing a conformational change that results in increasing

AT-III's activity. The activated AT-III then inactivates thrombin and other proteases involved in blood clotting. These factors include IIa (thrombin), Xa, IXa, XIa and XIIa. It is most active against thrombin and Xa. The rate of inactivation of these proteases by AT-III can increase by up to 1000-fold due to the binding of heparin. In addition, heparin increases the activity of heparin cofactor II, which also inhibits thrombin.

Heparin's onset is immediate and has a half-life of approximately 2.5 hours at doses of 300–400 USP units (U)/kg. It is provided in units, with 1 U, according to the US Pharmacopoeia, maintaining fluidity of 1 ml of citrated sheep plasma for 1 hour after recalcification.

## Dosing

Dosing of heparin can vary among institutions. The most common initial dose for CPB is 300–400 USP U/kg. Some centers base the initial dose on a bedside ex vivo heparin dose-response titration. Many institutions add heparin to the CPB priming solution at approximately the same concentration as that of the patient's bloodstream or as a fixed dose. Supplemental heparin doses are guided by monitoring of anticoagulation using the activated clotting time (ACT) or heparin concentration monitoring.

## Monitoring

The ACT is a funtional assay of heparin anticoagulation and is the most widely employed test. Most institutions use a level between 400 and 480 seconds as an acceptable ACT level at which to conduct CPB. Hypothermia, hemodilution, platelet function abnormalities and low fibrinogen are some of the factors that can prolong ACT, even in the setting of incomplete heparinization. ACT monitoring will be discussed in further detail under the section "Point-of-care testing."

## Heparin resistance

Heparin resistance is defined as failure to raise the ACT to expected levels despite an adequate dose and plasma concentration of heparin. Clinical conditions involving congenital or acquired AT-III deficiency are associated with heparin resistance. Hemodilution during CPB can decrease AT-III levels, though usually this does not result in heparin resistance because it is also associated with dilution of procoagulant factors. Prior treatment with heparin causes depletion or dysfunction of AT-III and this is the most likely reason that cardiac surgery patients will present with heparin resistance. Another cause of heparin resistance is the presence of large quantities of heparin-binding protein in the circulation, which binds to and inactivates heparin.

Administering additional heparin boluses of up to 600–800 USP U/kg may be necessary to obtain an ACT level sufficient for the conduct of CPB. Definitive treatment is aimed at increasing levels of AT-III. This can be done by administering fresh frozen plasma (FFP), which contains antithrombin; however, exposure to transfusion-borne infectious diseases is a risk. Supplemental AT-III concentrate is another alternative and provides greater protection against disease transmission than FFP. AT-III is also available in recombinant formulations, which have been used to treat congenital deficiency.

## Heparin-induced thrombocytopenia (HIT)

Heparin-induced thrombocytopenia (HIT) develops in 5% of patients receiving heparin and is categorized into two subtypes. The first type is generally mild and involves a transient decrease in platelet count. These patients can safely receive heparin for cardiac surgery. The second type occurs later in heparin therapy (5–14 days after administration) and is a more severe, immune-mediated decrease in the platelet count. Antibodies against the complex of platelet factor 4 (PF4) and heparin bind to platelets, activate the platelets and cause the resultant platelet count to drop precipitously. In the setting of endothelial injury, this enhancement in platelet activation predisposes to the formation of platelet clots (white clots) and thrombosis.

Heparin-induced thrombocytopenia is a clinicopathological syndrome and requires both clinical evidence (thrombocytopenia or thrombosis) and laboratory findings to confirm the diagnosis. Laboratory diagnosis can be made in two ways: functional assay or antibody-based assay. Functional tests detect heparin-dependent platelet activation in the presence of the patient's sera and UFH. The serotonin release assay (SRA) is considered the gold standard: when an affected patient's serum is exposed to heparin, an exaggerated reaction occurs and serotonin is released from dense granules. Using C-14-labeled serotonin the concentration released is then measurable. Other functional tests include the heparin-induced platelet activation assay (HIPAA) and the platelet-rich plasma (PRP) aggregation assay, which measure hyper-aggregability in response to heparin. Enzyme-linked immunological assays measure IgG, IgM or IgA antibodies that bind to the PF4/heparin complex.

The Seventh American College of Chest Physicians (ACCP) Conference on Antithrombotic and Thrombolytic Therapy resulted in the publication of evidence-based guidelines. Recommendations were made for patients undergoing cardiac surgery with previous HIT, as well as those with acute or subacute HIT. Grade 1 recommendations are strong and indicate that a high level of evidence suggests that the benefits of a particular intervention outweigh the risks, burden and costs. Grade 2 recommendations suggest that individual patients' or physicians' values may lead to different choices. Management of these patients can be summarized as follows: Patients with a history of HIT who are antibody negative and require cardiac surgery can receive unfractionated heparin. For patients with acute HIT who require cardiac surgery, the guideline developers recommend delaying surgery, if possible, until HIT antibodies are negative or using alternative anticoagulant approaches such as bivalrudin or hirudin. Combinations of unfractionated heparin and antiplatelet agents such as epoprostenol or tirofiban are also recommended.

## Alternatives to unfractionated heparin

### Low-molecular-weight heparin (LMWH)

Intravenously administered LMWH has a half-life at least twice as long as that of UFH and possibly several times as long for some LMWH compounds. Problems during CPB arise from the fact that protamine neutralization only reverses the factor IIa inhibition and leaves the predominant factor Xa inhibition intact. LMWH therapy also complicates heparin monitoring because activated partial thromboplastin time (APT) (and presumably ACT) is much less sensitive to Xa inhibition and will not accurately measure the full anticoagulant effect. Factor Xa inhibition can be measured, but not with a simple bedside test. LMWHs are not recommended for use in HIT patients

### Danaparoid

Danaparoid is a low-molecular-weight heparinoid with a long half-life (18–24 hours). It is a polysulfated glycosaminoglycan composed of heparan sulfate (84%), dermatan sulfate (12%)

and chondroitin sulfate (4%). There is a 30% cross-reactivity with heparin antibodies, which precludes its use in HIT patients. Monitoring is via anti-Xa levels and currently there is no antidote. It has been studied in CPB and has not been proven to be safe because of excess bleeding and thrombosis. Danaparoid is no longer available in the USA.

### Fibrinolytics

Ancrod (viprinex) is a defibrinogenating agent extracted from Malayan pit viper venom. Fibrinogen levels must be <500 mg/l prior to instituting CPB, which requires more than 12 hours after administering Ancrod to be achieved. Other disadvantages include no antidote, lack of monitoring and bleeding complications. Ancrod is not recommended for use in HIT patients.

### Direct thrombin inhibitors (DTIs)

These directly inhibit the procoagulant and prothrombotic actions of thrombin and do not require a cofactor. Their advantage is that they do not interact with or produce heparin-dependent antibodies. The main differences between the two types of thrombin inhibitors are listed in Table 4.1

- **Lepirudin** – This is a recombinant analogue of the anticoagulant hirudin produced in leech saliva. It has a short half-life of 80 minutes and is monitored via activated partial thromboplastin time (aPTT) or ACT and has no antidote. It can, however, be eliminated by hemofiltration. Lepirudin is metabolized by the kidney requiring dose adjustments in patients with renal insufficiency. The advantage is that it lacks cross-reactivity with heparin but antihirudin antibodies develop in as many as 60% of patients. Current evidence suggests that these antihirudin antibodies do not interfere with the anticoagulant activity of hirudin and their significance is unknown.
- **Argatroban** – This is a synthetic molecule derived from L-arginine and is widely used in patients with HIT who require percutaneous coronary intervention. Its half-life is 45–55 minutes, it lacks cross-reactivity with heparin antibodies and is monitored via the aPTT or ACT. There is no antidote. Argatroban is metabolized in the liver requiring dose adjustments in patients with moderate liver disease. Argatroban has not yet been approved for use in CPB. It is not available in the UK.
- **Bivalirudin** – This is a synthetic peptide based on the structure of hirudin. Its advantage is its short half-life of 25 minutes. It is monitored via the aPTT, ACT or ecarin clotting time, if available. The dose for CPB is a 1 mg/kg bolus followed by a 2.5 mg/kg/hour infusion. Bivalirudin is metabolized by proteolytic enzymes present in the blood and by the kidney. Only minor dose adjustments are necessary for patients with renal insufficiency. Multicenter trials have demonstrated it is not inferior to heparin when used in CPB. Currently, bivalirudin is widely used in cardiac catheterization laboratories as the anticoagulant for percutaneous coronary intervention, even in patients without HIT.

# "Reversal" of anticoagulation

## Heparin neutralization

Protamine is a naturally occurring polypeptide with multiple cationic sites, a "polycation" that binds and inactivates heparin.

**Table 4.1.** Key differences between direct thrombin inhibitors (DTIs) and indirect thrombin inhibitors

|  | Heparin | DTIs |
|---|---|---|
| Mode of action | Indirect | Direct |
| Cofactor needed | Yes – AT-III | No |
| Inhibits clot-bound thrombin | No | Yes |
| Activates platelets | Yes | No |
| Antigenicity | Yes | No – bivalirudin; Yes – hirudin |
| Antidote drug | Yes – protamine | No |

Several protamine dosing techniques have been utilized. The recommended dose range of protamine for heparin reversal is 1–1.3 mg protamine per 100 U of heparin. Other approaches include calculating the protamine dose based on the heparin dose–response curve generated by some automated systems such as the Hepcon (Medtronic Inc). Protamine must be administered slowly in order to prevent adverse hemodynamic effects such as hypotension.

Protamine reactions have been classified into three types. A Type I reaction may result from rapid administration resulting in decreases in both systemic and pulmonary arterial pressures, decreased preload and hypotension. The Type II reaction is immunological and is categorized as IIA anaphylaxis, IIB anaphylactoid and IIC non-cardiogenic pulmonary edema. Type III reactions are caused by heparin/protamine ionic complexes that can adhere in the pulmonary circulation and cause pulmonary vasoconstriction. This results in catastrophic pulmonary hypertension and resultant right heart failure.

Adequacy of neutralization should be assessed by repeating ACT 3–5 minutes after reversal.

## Alternatives to protamine

### Hexadimethrine

This synthetic polycation can be administered to patients who are allergic to protamine without adverse effects. However, when administered rapidly, hexadimethrine mimics the response to rapid administration of protamine because it forms complexes with heparin. Systemic hypotension, decreased systemic vascular resistance (SVR) and pulmonary vasoconstriction are among the adverse reactions seen. Following reports of renal toxicity, hexadimethrine was withdrawn from clinical use in the USA.

### Platelet factor 4 (PF4)

Platelets contain PF4, a potent antiheparin compound, on their surface, which utilizes lysine residues at it C-termini to neutralize heparin, rather than the electrostatic binding that occurs with protamine.

It is hypothesized that the cause of heparin-induced thrombocytopenia is an immunological reaction to the PF4/heparin complex.

### Methylene blue

This chemical dye binds electrostatically to heparin in a similar fashion to protamine. Large doses do not effectively restore the ACT to normal. An inhibitor of nitric oxide synthetase, methylene blue increases pulmonary and systemic vascular resistance at higher doses, making its use quite hazardous.

### Omit neutralization

Due to drug elimination, heparin will dissipate spontaneously with time with consequent decline in anticoagulation. This option may result in an increase in transfusion requirements, hemodynamic instability and consumptive coagulopathy as a result of hemorrhage and transfusions.

### Heparinase

Heparinase, an enzyme produced by the gram-negative *Flavobacterium*, hydrolyzes the heparin molecule into smaller inactive fragments. Some of these small fragments do possess the potential for some anti-Xa activity, thus the utility of heparinase in reversing heparin after CPB is limited.

## Monitoring anticoagulation status in the operating room

### Point-of-care testing (POC)

Point-of-care testing devices allow the monitoring of hemostasis at "the bedside" rather than sending specimens to a central laboratory facility. These instruments rapidly assess coagulation and/or platelet function to aid in providing appropriate targeted therapy. As a result there is a reduction in blood loss and transfusion, fewer complications and cost reduction.

The ACT is an automated variation of the Lee–White clotting time and is the most commonly used test to measure heparin anticoagulation. It uses an activator such as celite or kaolin to activate clotting, then measures the clotting time in a test tube or cartridge. Normal baseline ACT levels, without any heparin in the blood, should be between 80 and 140 seconds. For CPB, prolongation of the ACT to greater than 400 or 480 seconds is considered adequate, though this is highly debated. For off-pump coronary artery bypass operations (OPCAB), "partial heparinization" may be used in some centers whereby an ACT greater than 300 seconds is targeted. The Hemochron (International Technidyne Corp, Edison, NJ, USA) and the HemoTec ACT (Medtronic HemoTec, Parker, CO, USA) are two automated ACT devices used in the operating room.

During CPB the sensitivity of the ACT to heparin is altered by hemodilution and hypothermia. As a result ACT measurements do not correlate with heparin concentration or with antifactor Xa activity. The Hepcon HMS® analyzer (Medtronic Inc, Minneapolis, MN, USA) uses protamine titration assays to determine the blood heparin level. This device can also provide a dose–response curve for an individual patient and indicate how much heparin to administer in order to reach a specific targeted ACT before going onto CPB. In addition, it can be utilized for protamine dosing after CPB.

Other tests used less commonly to monitor heparin effectiveness during CPB are High Dose Thrombin Time (HiTT) (International Technidyne Inc, Edison, NJ, USA) and Heparin Management Test (HMT) Cascade Analyzer (Helena, Beaumont, TX, USA). HiTT measures the conversion of fibrinogen to fibrin by thrombin and, unlike ACT, HiTT is not affected by hemodilution, hypothermia or aprotinin. The Cascade® coagulation analyzer can measure prothrombin time (PT), aPTT and HiTT levels in whole blood at the point of care.

# Tests of platelet function

## Thromboelastography (TEG)

Thromboelastography measures the viscoelastic properties of blood as it is induced to clot under a low shear environment resembling sluggish venous flow. The patterns of change in shear–elasticity enable the determination of the kinetics of clot formation and clot growth and provide information about clot strength and stability. The strength and stability of the clot provides information about the ability of the clot to cause hemostasis effectively, while the kinetics determine the adequacy of quantitative factors available for clot formation.

There are four major parameters to the TEG tracing, which measure different stages of clot development: R, K, alpha angle and MA (maximal amplitude). In addition, clot lysis indices are measured as the amplitude at 30 and 60 minutes after MA (LY30 and LY60) (see Figure 4.2). Normal values vary depending on the type of activator used.

- **R value** – This is a measure of clotting time from the start of the bioassay to the initial fibrin formation. R time can be prolonged by coagulation factor deficiencies, anticoagulation, severe thrombocytopenia and hypofibrinogenemia. R time can be shortened in hypercoagulability states.
- **K value** – This represents clot kinetics, measuring the speed to reach a specific level of clot strength. It is the time from beginning of clot formation (the end of R time) until the amplitude reaches 20 mm. K time can be prolonged by coagulation factor deficiencies, hypofibrinogenemia, thrombocytopenia and thrombocytopathy. It is shortened in hypercoagulable states.
- **Alpha angle** – This is the angle between the line in the middle of the TEG tracing and the line tangential to the developing "body" of the TEG tracing. The alpha angle represents the acceleration (kinetics) of fibrin build up and cross-linking (clot strengthening). It is increased in hypercoagulable states and decreased in thrombocytopenia and hypofibringenemia.
- **MA** – This is the maximum amplitude reflecting the ultimate strength of the clot, which depends on platelet number and function and platelet interactions with fibrin. It is increased in hypercoagulable states and decreased in thrombocytopenia, thrombocytopathy and hypofibrinogenemia.
- **Lysis** – Indices measured by the TEG include LY30 and LY60. These are the percentage ratio of the amplitude at 30 and 60 minutes after MA to the MA itself. LY30 or LY60 are increased in states of fibrinolysis.

## Other POC tests of platelet function

Sonoclot is an alternative test to TEG of the viscoelastic properties of blood. Sonoclot uses an ultrasonic vibrational method to stimulate clot formation.

The newest group of POC platelet function tests were specifically designed to measure agonist-induced platelet-mediated hemostasis. These monitoring systems include the VerifyNow (Accumetrics, San Diego, CA, USA), the Clot Signature Analyzer (CSA, Xylum, Scarsdale, NY, USA), the Platelet Function Analyzer, PFA-100 (Dade Behring, Miami, FL, USA) and Plateletworks (Helena Laboratories, Beaumont, TX, USA) (see Table 4.2). The CSA is not currently FDA approved.

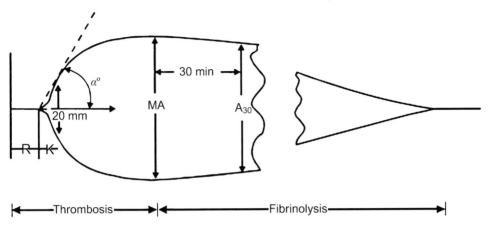

**Figure 4.2.** Normal TEG trace (refer to text for details of abbreviations).

**Table 4.2.** POC devices to assess platelet function

| Instrument | Mechanism/agonist | Clinical utility |
|---|---|---|
| Thromboelastograph® | Viscoelastic/thrombin, ADP, arachidonic acid (AA) | Post-CPB, liver transplant, pediatrics, obstetrics, drug efficacy |
| Sonoclot® | Viscoelastic/thrombin | Post-CPB, liver transplant |
| PlateletWorks® | Platelet count ratio/ADP, AA, collagen | Post-CPB, drug therapy |
| PFA-100® | In vitro bleeding time/ADP, epinephrine | von Willebrand's disease, congenital disorder, aspirin therapy, |
| post-CPB | | |
| VerifyNow® | Agglutination/thrombin receptor agonist peptide (TRAP), AA, ADP | Drug therapy |
| Clot Signature Analyzer® | Shear-induced in vitro bleeding time/collagen | Post-CPB, drug effects |
| Whole blood aggregometry | Electrical impedance/many | Post-CPB |

# Coagulation disorders after CPB

Persistent bleeding after CPB is multifactorial. It is usually associated with long bypass times (>2 hours) as a result of which platelet dysfunction, hemodilution, protein activation/consumption and fibrinolysis occur. Prompt diagnostic and therapeutic action is necessary to avoid impaired hemodynamics due to hemorrhage.

## Platelet abnormalities

Thrombocytopenia can occur after CPB due to dilution of blood volume with the extracorporeal circuit volume and platelet consumption or sequestration. Platelet function impairment is considered to be the main hemostatic defect during CPB. Platelet dysfunction occurs from contact with the extracorporeal surfaces, hypothermia, down-regulation of receptors and by exposure to heparin and protamine. In addition, patients on antithrombotic medications preoperatively can have platelet dysfunction that becomes significantly exaggerated after CPB. Many patients taking aspirin or other platelet-inhibiting drugs regularly cannot discontinue therapy within 7 days of surgery and unfortunately no antidote can correct the platelet defect. These patients have a very difficult bleeding diathesis that often requires multiple transfusions and/or pro-coagulant factor therapy.

## Systemic inflammatory response syndrome

Contact of blood with the CPB circuit results in the systemic inflammatory response syndrome (SIRS), which is characterized by the activation of the kallikrein–bradykinin system, complement, coagulation pathways and fibrinolysis. SIRS may cause disseminated intravascular coagulation (DIC) by aggravating consumption of coagulation factors (see Chapter 11).

## Heparin rebound

This phenomenon may be observed after apparent adequate reversal of heparinization and may be explained by a redistribution either of protamine to peripheral compartments or of peripherally bound heparin to the central compartment. Treatment is with small incremental doses of protamine.

## Hypothermia

Hemostasis is impaired by hypothermia in many ways including: sequestration of platelets, transient platelet dysfunction, activation of a specific heparin-like inhibitor of Xa, slowing of the enzymatic reactions involved in the coagulation cascade and accentuation of fibrinolysis.

## Fibrinolysis

The CPB circuit contains a large surface of thrombogenic material and, despite clinically adequate doses and blood concentrations of heparin, activation of coagulation pathways is accompanied by persistent fibrinolytic activity causing consumption of coagulation factors.

## Other causes

Hemodilution, liberal use of cardiotomy suction and prolonged CPB all further aggravate coagulopathy.

# Prevention of bleeding

## Antifibrinolytic agents

- The synthetic antifibrinolytic agents ε-aminocaparoic acid (EACA) and tranexamic acid (TA) bind to lysine binding sites in both plasminogen and plasmin and produce a structural change. This prevents the conversion of plasminogen to plasmin and also prevents the activation of plasmin. Minimization of plasmin activity inhibits fibrin degradation, decreases the formation of fibrin degradation products (FDPs) and decreases lysis of existing clots. It is these FDPs that inhibit platelet function, so the lysine analogue anti-fibrinolytic agents also have an indirect effect in preserving platelet function. Dosing of these agents is highly variable and is dependent on institution and country. Typical regimens are given below:

· EACA 100–150 mg/kg bolus, followed by infusion at 10–15 mg/kg/hour, or 4–6 g bolus, followed by infusion at 1 g/hour; and
· TA: 10–50 mg/kg bolus, followed by infusion at 1–15 mg/kg/hour, or 5 g bolus, followed by repeat boluses to total of 15 g.

• Aprotinin, a serine protease inhibitor isolated from bovine lung that inhibits several enzymatic activators of coagulation including plasmin and kallikrein. Its action on kallikrein leads to the inhibition of the formation of factor XIIa. As a result, both the intrinsic pathway of coagulation and fibrinolysis are inhibited. Its action on plasmin independently slows fibrinolysis. Dosing – Full Dose Regimen (Hammersmith Protocol): a test dose of 10 000 kallikrein-inhibiting units (KIU) should be administered followed 10 minutes later by 2 million KIU as a bolus, 2 million KIU added to the pump prime and 500 000 KIU/hour as an infusion. As of November 2007, worldwide marketing of aprotinin has been suspended after publication of observational studies and the randomized Canadian BART ("Blood Conservation using Antifibrinolytics: A Randomized Trial") trial. The BART trial was an independent randomized control trial conducted in high-risk cardiac patients that was halted after data revealed reduced bleeding as well as an increase in all-cause mortality in patients receiving aprotinin compared to those receiving either aminocaproic acid or tranexemic acid.

• Heparin and protamine dosing: ACT should return to baseline following administration of protamine; additional doses of protamine (25–50 mg) may be necessary. Reheparinization (heparin rebound) after apparent adequate reversal may be explained by a redistribution either of protamine to peripheral compartments or of peripherally bound heparin to the central compartment.

• Desmopressin is an analogue of vasopressin that releases von Willebrand factor (VWF) from normal endothelial cells and is used in the treatment of hemophilia. Factor VIII coagulant activity increases 2- to 20-fold in addition to an increase in factor XII levels. Desmopressin has been beneficial to subgroups of patients, such as cirrhotic and uremic patients, undergoing cardiac surgery. It affords no hemostatic benefit to patients taking aspirin prior to cardiac surgery and is not recommended as a prophylactic hemostatic agent for patients undergoing elective cardiac surgery. It may also be used to augment the function of exogenous transfused platelets.

• Use of non-pharmacological strategies:

· The use of heparin-bonded CPB circuits makes the extracorporeal circuit more biocompatible thus effectively reducing the proinflammatory aspects of CPB.
· Some clinicians advocate the use of a reduced heparin dose in conjunction with heparin-bonded circuits to decrease postoperative blood loss and transfusion requirements.

# Management of the bleeding patient

Determining the cause of bleeding quickly is vital to expedite treatment of the bleeding patient. Surgical causes of bleeding generally present with generous chest tube drainage early after operation. Non-surgical causes of bleeding usually manifest as a generalized ooze.

Hypothermia ($<35°C$) accentuates hemostatic defects and should be corrected. The administration of platelets and coagulation factors should generally be guided by additional coagulation studies, but empirical therapy may be necessary when such tests are not readily available, or following massive transfusion.

If oozing continues despite adequate surgical hemostasis and the ACT is normal or the heparin–protamine titration assay shows no residual heparin, thrombocytopenia or platelet dysfunction is most likely. Both defects are recognized complications of CPB. Platelet transfusion may be necessary and should be given to maintain the platelet count above $100\,000/\mu l$. Significant depletion of coagulation factors, particularly factors V and VIII, during CPB is less commonly responsible for bleeding but should be treated with fresh frozen plasma; both the prothrombin time and partial thromboplastin time are usually prolonged in such instances. Hypofibrinogenemia (fibrinogen level $<100$ mg/dl or a prolonged thrombin time without residual heparin) should be treated with cryoprecipitate. Desmopressin (DDAVP), $0.3\,\mu g/kg$ (intravenously slowly over 20 minutes), can increase the activity of factors VIII and XII and the von Willebrand factor by releasing them from the vascular endothelium. DDAVP may be effective in reversing qualitative platelet defects in some patients, but is not recommended for routine use.

Accelerated fibrinolysis may occasionally be encountered following CPB and should be treated with ε-aminocaproic acid (5 g followed by 1 g/hour) or tranexamic acid (10 mg/kg), if not already being given; the diagnosis should be confirmed by elevated fibrin degradation products ($>32$ mg/ml), or evidence of clot lysis on thromboelastography.

Recombinant factor VIIa (rFVIIa, NovoSeven) is a vitamin K-dependent glycoprotein that promotes hemostasis by activating the extrinsic pathway of the coagulation cascade. Tissue factor-bearing cells present tissue factor to rFVIIa. This complex can activate factor X to factor Xa, as well as factor IX to IXa. Factor Xa, in complex with other factors, then converts prothrombin to thrombin, which leads to the formation of a hemostatic plug by converting fibrinogen to fibrin and thereby inducing local hemostasis. This process can also occur on the surface of activated platelets. rFVIIa has been approved for use in hemophiliacs who are resistant to factor VIII concentrates. Numerous reports have been published in cardiac surgery as an "off-label" treatment option in patients with probable or identifiable coagulation defects or as a rescue therapy in hemorrhagic patients refractory to other treatments.

## Transfusion and the use of algorithms

Point-of-care testing in conjunction with transfusion algorithms can reduce both transfusion requirements and blood loss. Many transfusion algorithms have been published and demonstrate a successful reduction in bleeding and transfusion requirements in high-risk cardiac surgical patients. Most of these transfusion algorithms utilize the thromboelastogram, others use point of care PT and international normalized ratio (INR) testing, and others use tests of platelet function and number. Any combination of tests that examines the presumed defects incurred during CPB will accomplish the same goal – the reduction in the transfusion of blood products by more rational and specific guidance of that transfusion therapy.

Hemostasis and bleeding in conjunction with cardiac surgery is a multifactorial problem. The defects that occur are dynamic in origin and knowledge of physiological responses to CPB continue to evolve.

# Suggested Further Reading

- Despotis GJ, Joist JH, Goodnough LT. Monitoring of hemostasis in cardiac surgical patients: impact of point-of-care testing on blood loss and transfusion outcomes. *Clinl Chem* 1997; **43**: 1684–96.

- Raivio P, Suojaranta-Ylinen R, Kuitunen AH. Recombinant factor VIIa in the treatment of postoperative hemorrhage after cardiac surgery. *Ann Thorac Surg* 2005; **80**: 66–71.

- Rochon AG, Shore-Lesserson L. Coagulation monitoring. *Anesthesiol Clin North Am* 2006; **24**(4): 839–56.

- Romagnoli S, Bevilacqua S, Gelsomino S, *et al*. Small-dose recombinant activated factor VII (NovoSeven) in cardiac surgery. *Anesth Analg* 2006; **102**: 1320–6.

- Shore-Lesserson L. Coagulation monitoring. In Kaplan JA, ed. *Kaplan's Cardiac Anesthesia*, 5th ed. Philadelphia: Elsevier Saunders; 2006: 557–82.

- Shore-Lesserson L, Horrow JC, Gravlee GP. Coagulation management during and after cardiopulmonary bypass. In Kaplan JA, Reich DL, Lake CL, Konstadt SN, eds. *A Practical Approach to Cardiac Anesthesia*, 4th ed. Philadelphia: Lippincott Williams and Wilkins; 2008: 494–515.

- Spiess BD, Gillies BSA, Chandler W, Verrier E. Changes in transfusion therapy and reexploration rate after institution of a blood management program in cardiac surgical patients. *J Cardiothorac Vasc Anesth* 1995; **9**: 168–73.

- Spiess BD, Horrow JC, Kaplan JA. Transfusion medicine and coagulation disorders. In Kaplan JA, ed. *Kaplan's Cardiac Anesthesia*, 5th ed. Philadelphia: Elsevier Saunders; 2006: 937–84.

- Spiess BD, Tuman KJ, McCarthy RJ, DeLaria GA, Schillo R, Ivankovich AD. Thrombelastography as an indicator of post-cardiopulmonary bypass coagulopathies. *J Clin Monit* 1987; **3**: 25–30.

- The Seventh American College of Chest Physicians (ACCP). Conference on Antithrombotic and Thrombolytic Therapy: evidence-based guidelines. *Chest* 2004; **126**: 3(suppl).

- Warkentin TE, Greinacher A. Heparin-induced thrombocytopenia: recognition, treatment, and prevention: The 7th ACCP Conference on Antithrombotic & Thrombolytic Therapy. *Chest* 2004; **126**: 311S–337S.

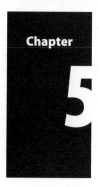

# Conduct of cardiopulmonary bypass

Betsy Evans, Helen Dunningham and John Wallwork

Chapter
5

The pump is your friend!
*Caves, 1976*

Cardiopulmonary bypass is an incredible facility when used correctly by the team of surgeon, anesthetist and perfusionist. A comprehensive understanding of the physiology of CPB is essential for optimum benefit, together with knowledge of the risks, limitations and potential adverse effects if used incorrectly. The management of CPB involves a multi-disciplinary approach with coordinated actions and precise communication being crucial for a safe, effective outcome.

Before each case the conduct of CPB should be planned. All members of the team need to be aware of the intended method for cannulation, the systemic and myocardial temperatures required during surgery, the technique of myocardial protection to be used, whether deep hypothermic circulatory arrest (DHCA) will be required and the most appropriate sites for monitoring during CPB.

Prior to assembly of the CPB circuit, patient demographic data and information relating to physiological and pathological status are required to enable selection of equipment tailored to the patient's needs.

## Arterial cannulation

The arterial cannula is usually the narrowest part of the CPB circuit with resultant high resistance, pressure gradients, high velocity jets and turbulence. The effect of jets on the interior wall of the aorta can lead to arterial dissection, embolization and flow disturbances in head and neck vessels.

The "performance index" of an arterial cannula is the pressure gradient versus the outer diameter at any given flow. The narrowest portion of the catheter that enters the aorta should be as short as safely possible and the diameter should then gradually increase in size to minimize the gradient. Pressure gradients greater than 100 mmHg can cause excessive hemolysis and should be avoided. Many different types of cannulae are available and are discussed further in Chapter 1.

"Straight" arterial cannulae are the most commonly used, with some having a flange to allow secure fixation to the aorta with minimal tip within the vessel. The straight design allows non-turbulent blood flow through the cannula, but results in a single jet of blood, which can cause damage to the aortic wall. The straight nature of the cannula means that the flow direction is reliant on the surgical placement. In addition to direct placement in the aorta these cannulae can be used for peripheral (e.g. femoral or axillary) arterial cannulation or within a graft.

Right-angled cannulae have been designed to allow the blood flow jet to be directed around the aortic arch, assuming correct placement. Right-angled "diffusion" cannulae, with

*Cardiopulmonary Bypass,* ed. S. Ghosh, F. Falter and D. J. Cook. Published by Cambridge University Press.
© Cambridge University Press 2009.

diffusion holes and a sealed end, may attenuate the damaging jet effect by changing the flow characteristics into the aorta. However, concern has been expressed regarding increased hemolysis due to the more turbulent flow effect through the cannula. These cannulae are not suitable for femoral placement.

## Connection to patient

Usually arterial inflow is directed into the ascending aorta. The advantages of this site are:

- ease;
- safety;
- single incision;
- size of cannula not usually limited by vessel diameter; and
- no risk of limb ischemia.

The site for cannulation in the ascending aorta is traditionally determined by intraoperative palpation for calcific atherosclerotic plaques; however, newer techniques such as transesophageal echocardiography (TOE) or epivascular ultrasonic scanning are now being used to determine plaque-free areas for cannulation. If significant atherosclerosis is present such that aortic cannulation and cross-clamping is deemed unsafe, because of the risk of stroke due to dislodgement and embolization of atherosclerotic material, femoral arterial cannulation should be considered. It must be noted that retrograde perfusion via femoral arterial cannulation is not without risk of embolization of atheroma and in such instances subclavian or innominate arterial cannulation may be preferable. In the event of a totally calcified "porcelain aorta," alternative strategies that minimize aortic handling such as OPCAB surgery or the use of DHCA may be appropriate.

Prior to insertion of the aortic cannula, the chosen site is prepared with placement of opposing purse-string sutures and clearance of the adventitial tissue within the boundaries of these sutures. With the mean arterial pressure controlled at between 70 and 80 mmHg, to avoid excessive bleeding or trauma to the aorta, particularly dissection, a full-thickness incision is made in the aortic wall through which the aortic cannula is passed. Only 1–2 cm of the cannula tip is advanced and directed towards the arch to avoid inadvertent cannulation of the head and neck vessels or dissection of the posterior wall of the aorta. The aortic cannula is immediately de-aired by allowing blood to fill the tubing, which is then clamped and secured with the purse-string sutures, prior to connecting to the arterial inflow circuitry of the CPB machine. During connection to the circuit it is essential to ensure that no air is present at the connection site. When the connection is complete the perfusionist will inform the surgeon of the "swing" on the arterial pressure line and the pressure within the system to confirm correct intraluminal placement of the cannula.

## Complications of aortic root cannulation

If air is introduced into the aortic line during aortic cannulation, the line must be disconnected from the aortic cannula and the air aspirated prior to reconnection. If gross air embolism is noted in the aortic line during established CPB, it may be possible for the perfusionist to remove the air via recirculation lines in the CPB circuit with only a brief interruption to pump flow. If gross systemic air embolism occurs, de-airing of the cerebral circulation must be attempted. With the patient in the Trendelenberg position CPB is terminated followed by removal of the arterial cannula from the aorta, leaving the purse-string sutures loose. The arterial line is filled and then inserted into the SVC. Retrograde perfusion to the cerebral circulation via the SVC using low flow rates (1–2 l/minute), at a blood temperature of 20°C, enables de-airing of the cerebral circulation back to the aorta. During this de-airing process the perfusionist should re-prime the circuit, followed by the surgeon re-cannulating the ascending aorta and recommencement of CPB at 28°C until surgery is completed. CPB should be discontinued at a core temperature of 35°C. The use of relative hypothermia increases the solubility of gaseous emboli and may reduce the extent of cerebral injury.

Further potential complications of aortic root cannulation are summarized in Table 5.1.

## Peripheral arterial cannulation

Indications for the use of peripheral arterial cannulation not only include aortic aneurysm or an aorta that is not suitable for cannulation due to calcification, but also to establish CPB in anticipation of complications arising from redo-sternotomy. Increasingly, peripheral cannulation is also being used to enable "limited access," minimally invasive surgery. Femoral cannulation renders it necessary to use smaller size cannulae, with consequent higher pressure

**Table 5.1.** Complications of aortic root cannulation

Inability to introduce the cannula
- adventitia occluding the incision site
- inadequate incision size
- atheromatous plaque within aortic wall

Intramural placement

Embolization of atheromatous plaque

Air embolization on connection to the circuit

Persistent bleeding around cannula

Malposition of tip towards aortic valve or into arch vessels

Dissection of aorta

Kink in circuit

Inadequate size leading to high pressure and low flow generation

Aneurysm formation at site of cannulation at later stage

**Table 5.2.** Complications of peripheral cannulation

Trauma to vessel

Retrograde arterial dissection with retroperitoneal hemorrhage or extension of dissection to aortic root

Thrombosis or embolism

Hemorrhage

Limb ischemia (can be reduced by using an end to side polytetrafluoroethane (PTFE) graft sutured to the vessel)

Malperfusion of cerebral and systemic circulation as a result of cannulation of the false lumen of an aortic dissection

Lymph fistula or lymphocele

Infection

Late vascular stenosis

gradients, jet effects and possibly lower flow rates; this may be improved by cannulation of iliac arteries.

Axillary cannulation is usually employed in cases of ascending aortic dissection, to avoid the risk of inadvertent retrograde perfusion via the false lumen of the dissection, which can occur with femoral cannulation in these patients. The axillary artery is less likely than the femoral artery to have atherosclerotic disease or dissection and also has a good collateral flow, with less risk of limb ischemia. In addition to these benefits it provides antegrade flow, with reduced risk of cerebral embolization. Direct arterial cannulation or indirect cannulation via a side graft can be used to access the axillary artery; side graft placement and cannulation is usually preferable to direct cannulation.

The potential complications of peripheral cannulation are summarized in Table 5.2.

## Venous cannulation and drainage

Venous blood inflow to the CPB circuit is usually achieved by gravity drainage, using the "siphon" effect, but earlier CPB circuits used suction to aid venous drainage; in pediatric cases, drainage is still often aided by applying suction to the venous lines. Gravity siphoning as the means of obtaining adequate drainage relies on:

(1)     no air being present in the tubing between the patient and the pump, otherwise an "air-lock" develops and drainage stops; and

(2)     the venous reservoir being kept below the level of the patient's thorax.

The degree of venous drainage is determined by the patient's central venous pressure (CVP), the difference in height between the patient and the top of the blood level in the venous reservoir and resistance exerted by the circuit (cannulae, lines and connectors). The CVP is influenced by intravascular volume and venous compliance; which is in turn influenced by sympathetic tone. This is largely dependent on the extent of inflammatory response to CPB and by drugs used perioperatively.

Excessive drainage may cause the veins to collapse around the cannulae with intermittent reduction in venous drainage and the potential for generation of gaseous emboli in the circuit; a phenomenon referred to as "cavitation."

## Types and sizes of venous cannulae (see Chapter 1)

The cannula tip is the narrowest component in the venous circuit and therefore the limiting factor for venous drainage. The appropriate size is selected based on the flow characteristics of the cannula (detailed in the manufacturer's guidelines) and the required flow for the patient based on cardiac index. One third of total flow is derived from SVC drainage and two-thirds from IVC drainage.

Cannulae can be divided according to three main criteria:

- single versus two-stage (cavo-atrial);
- straight or angled; and
- metal or plastic.

## Connection to the patient

This is usually achieved by right atrial (RA) cannulation. There are three basic approaches:

- **Single** – A cannula is passed through the RA appendage: this route is advantageous because it is quick and the least traumatic, but it is most sensitive to changes in position of the heart and venous drainage can be impaired with cardiac retraction. This technique cannot be used if the right heart is to be opened.

- **Cavo-atrial** – This uses a "two-stage" cannula with a wider proximal portion, with side holes, which lies in the RA and a narrow extension, with end and side holes, extending into the IVC. This cannula is typically inserted through the right atrial appendage and cannot be used if the right heart is to be opened.
- **Bicaval** – Purse-string sutures are placed on the posterior–inferior RA wall and the RA appendage to enable direct cannulation of the IVC and SVC, respectively. Tapes or snares are passed around the vessels with the cannulae in place to ensure that the patient's entire venous return flows into the CPB circuit, preventing air from entering the venous lines when opening the RA, or blood leaking past the cannulae into the RA; this is referred to as caval occlusion or total CPB and is the technique of choice if the right heart is to be opened.

It should be noted that the right heart may need to be vented via the pulmonary artery to prevent RV distension due to return of blood into the RA via the coronary sinus. Occasionally high SVC or even innominate vein cannulation may be required to facilitate the operation, for example, resection of an RA tumor mass or during operations needing access to the SVC such as some heart transplant or heart–lung transplant procedures (Domino heart).

In clinical practice most CABG and AVR surgery is performed with venous drainage via cavo-atrial cannulation. This usually provides adequate drainage as long as right heart decompression is constantly monitored and communication is maintained between the team regarding venous return, with the necessary adjustments of cannulae position during the operation to accommodate changes in heart position.

Air entry into the venous side of the circuit may lead to an "air lock," causing obstruction of venous drainage, or to systemic gaseous microemboli. The most common reason for air entry into the system is failure to seal the site around the cannulae adequately. Care must therefore be taken to ensure that purse-string sutures are air-tight, especially if vacuum-assisted venous drainage is being used.

## Peripheral venous cannulation

This is usually performed via the femoral or iliac veins and is used in the following instances:

- unstable patients for emergency establishment of CPB prior to sternotomy or anesthetic induction;
- selected redo-surgery: to provide controlled conditions during sternotomy and exposure of the heart;
- aortic surgery;
- thoracic surgery;
- minimal access surgery; and
- extracorporeal membrane oxygenation (ECMO).

The essential requirement is for adequate venous drainage and subsequent flow rates for CPB. With peripheral cannulation this is achieved by using as large a cannula as possible, and passing the cannula into the RA (often using TOE guidance). Vacuum-assisted venous drainage is advantageous under these circumstances, given the smaller cannula diameter and increased resistance from the cannula length.

Possible complications associated with venous cannulation are listed in Table 5.3.

**Table 5.3.** Complications of venous cannulation

Low cardiac output due to compression of the heart during IVC purse-string placement

Damage to SVC/IVC/right pulmonary artery whilst passing tapes around cavae

Reduction in cardiac output prior to commencement of CPB when cannulae are in place

Atrial dysrhythmia

Malpositioning of cannula tip

- SVC cannula into the azygos vein
- IVC cannula into the hepatic vein
- RA cannula into LA in the presence of an atrial secundum defect

RA trauma and bleeding from cannulation sites

SVC or IVC laceration on manipulation of cannulated RA

Narrowing of cavae after decannulation and closure of purse-string suture

Low venous return during CPB

- Kinks in circuit with obstruction of line
- Reduced venous pressure – volume or pressure related (drugs, anesthetic agents)
- Air lock
- Inadequate height of patient above CPB venous reservoir
- Inadequate size of cannula

# Cardiotomy suction

During cardiac surgery "shed" blood often needs to be suctioned from the operative field to maintain visibility for surgery and from cardiac chambers to prevent distension of the heart. After systemic heparinization, shed blood is salvaged through designated "cardiotomy" suckers and vents and collected in the reservoir for re-circulation within the CPB circuit.

Cardiotomy suction is most commonly generated by use of a roller pump, requiring repeated adjustment of pump flow rate by the perfusionist and sucker position by the surgeon due to the degree of negative pressure that can develop at the sucker tip leading to hemolysis of red blood cells and occasional occlusion of the sucker.

In extreme cases of hemorrhage, after heparinization with the arterial cannula in situ, the patient can be placed on "sucker bypass"; the shed blood in the operative field provides venous return to the CPB circuit until formal venous cannulation can be secured.

## Adverse effects of cardiotomy suction

Blood suctioned from the surgical field is highly "activated" with regard to coagulation factors, fibrinolytic mediators, leukocytes and platelets. It is a major source of hemolysis, microparticles, fat, cellular aggregates, inflammatory mediators (tumor necrosis factor alpha (TNF-$\alpha$), interleukin-6 (IL-6), C3a) and endotoxins, and a cause of platelet injury and loss. A potential determinant of injury caused by cardiotomy suction is the amount of room air coaspirated with the blood.

Commonly used strategies to reduce the side effects of cardiotomy suction are shown in Table 5.4.

**Table 5.4.** Strategies to reduce the side effects of cardiotomy suction

| |
|---|
| Hemostasis throughout operation to minimize shed blood |
| Minimize aspiration of air through the cardiotomy suction by |
| •     avoidance of high negative pressures |
| •     slow rates of suction |
| •     not sucking the surgical field dry |
| •     keeping the suction tip under level of blood |
| Filtration of cardiotomy suction blood (leukocyte depletion) |
| Cell salvage blood instead of cardiotomy suction |
| Off-pump surgery |

# Venting the heart

The left side of the heart receives blood whilst on CPB from bronchial arteries and Thebesian veins and the right heart from the coronary sinus and "leakage" around venous cannulae. As the ventricles are unable to eject this blood during the period of arrest, a vent must be placed to protect the heart from distension. Ventricular distension is undesirable because excessive myocardial stretching increases myocardial oxygen demand and impairs subendocardial perfusion.

On occasions, blood can return from abnormal sources. These include:

- left-sided SVC;
- patent ductus arteriosus (PDA);
- atrial septal defect/ventricular septal defect;
- anomalous venous drainage;
- aortic regurgitation; and
- systemic to pulmonary shunt.

## Venting the left heart

The left ventricle needs to be vented if it is filling from any source but not ejecting. It will fill primarily because of aortic insufficiency, or during cardioplegia administration. Venting:

- prevents distension of the ventricle;
- reduces myocardial re-warming;
- prevents ejection of air; and
- provides a bloodless surgical field.

Surgical inspection and palpation of the LV to monitor the degree of distension is crucial on commencing CPB, during aortic cross-clamping and during initial administration of cardioplegia. The use of a left atrial pressure monitoring line and pulmonary artery (PA) catheter can help detect moderate LV distension, which is sometimes a subtle finding.

## Venting the right heart

The venous cannulae effectively vent the right side of the heart, keeping it empty of blood except for any "leakage" past the cannula; this can be minimized by using bicaval cannulation and caval snares. When antegrade cardioplegia is administered, releasing the caval snare will permit venting of cardioplegia solution returning via the coronary sinus to the right heart.

Placement of a pulmonary arterial vent will keep the right ventricle empty of fluid. Persistent left SVC requires additional drainage of the coronary sinus or RA.

## Venting methods

Venting can be achieved via:

- the aortic root cardioplegia cannula – this method does not allow venting during cardioplegia administration;
- the right superior pulmonary vein – a vent is passed into the left atrium and through the mitral valve into the LV;
- the left ventricular apex; and
- the pulmonary artery – this may not be effective at venting the LV when there is aortic regurgitation with a competent mitral valve.

It must be remembered that venting the heart is not without complications. These can be immediate or delayed. "Steal" of systemic perfusion may occur if excessive venting of the heart is employed in the presence of aortic regurgitation. Systemic air embolism may occur when the vent is inserted or removed. Bleeding can occur from the vent site, particularly if an LV apical vent is used. Later complications of venting include stenosis of the pulmonary vein or pulmonary artery, or aneurysm of the LV apex, depending on the vent site used.

## General management of CPB

Before commencing CPB the perfusionists must have completed a series of "checks" as detailed in Chapter 2.

## Transition of patient onto CPB

The general sequence of events entailed in commencing CPB is described below and summarized at the end of this chapter in Appendix 5A:

- The patient must be systemically heparinized with confirmation of adequate anticoagulation (ACT >400 s). ACT targets vary among institutions and are the subject of much practical and academic debate. Heparin resistance must be considered if a therapeutic ACT cannot be achieved despite additional systemic boluses of heparin. Antithrombin III (AT-III) deficiency can be treated by giving AT-III-rich blood products such as FFP or AT-III concentrate. Repeat ACT should result in an elevated reading without the need for further heparin.
- Recirculation of CPB prime through the circuit to ensure that perfusate is warm and lines are air free.
- Division of the arterial and venous lines after clamps are applied at the patient and pump ends.
- The arterial line is connected to the aortic cannula, enabling rapid transfusion, if required, directly from the pump. During connection to the arterial line, the arterial cannula is allowed to bleed out slowly from the patient and the CPB prime is simultaneously advanced up the arterial line to ensure an air-free connection.

- Release of the aortic line clamp, after which the pressure "swing" is confirmed to indicate correct positioning of the aortic cannula.
- Retrograde autologous priming may be used to reduce the effect of hemodilution due to large prime volumes in the CPB circuit. The cardiotomy reservoir is primed to a minimal level and the patient's arterial blood is used to fill the circuit to a "safe" level after placement of the arterial cannula (this is approximately 400 ml). Hemodynamic consequences of this technique need to be considered for each patient. This technique is discussed in more detail in Chapter 3.
- The venous cannula is connected to the venous line.
- CPB is initiated, after instructions from the surgeon, by the perfusionist releasing the arterial line clamp and slowly transfusing the patient with the CPB prime. Arterial flow should be unobstructed and with an initial line pressure of less than 100 mmHg. The perfusionist must confirm that the oxygenator gases and CPB safety alarms are switched on prior to CPB.
- The venous clamp is gradually released after confirmation that the arterial line is unobstructed; the patient's venous blood is then diverted into the circuit. The right heart should decompress with a fall in CVP to less than 5 mmHg.
- A period of 1–2 minutes of transition occurs whilst the perfusionist gradually increases the rate of arterial flow and venous return to the heart is reduced. The arterial pressure changes to a non-pulsatile waveform. Pulsatility whilst on CPB indicates aortic valve insufficiency, inadequate venous drainage or excessive bronchial venous return into the heart.
- Most CPB systems generate non-pulsatile flow, but some do have computerized configurations to allow for pulsatile flow generation. Alternatively, pulsatile flow can be generated via an intra-aortic balloon pump, if in situ. There are many reported benefits of pulsatile flow such as increased renal, cerebral and myocardial perfusion together with a reduction of the stress response to CPB. However, in clinical studies, the conclusions are equivocal.
- Cooling of the patient, if required by the surgeon, is commenced once the patient is on full flow and adequate decompression of the heart is confirmed.

## Recommended flow rates for CPB

The primary requirement for CPB is to provide a systemic $O_2$ delivery ($DO_2$) that is sufficient to meet systemic $O_2$ demand ($VO_2$). In contrast to the intact native circulation, $DO_2$ is not controlled by reflex mechanisms, but by the perfusionist. During CPB whole body $DO_2$ is a function of pump flow and arterial oxygen content, the latter being primarily determined by the HCT. The major determinants of $VO_2$ are temperature and level of anesthesia.

Oxygen consumption ($VO_2$) can be calculated using the Fick equation:

$$VO_2 = Q(C_{(a-v)})O_2$$
$VO_2$ = minute oxygen consumption (ml/minute)
$Q$ = cardiac output (l/minute)
$$(C_{(a-v)})O_2 = 1.34 \times Hb + P_{(a-v)}O_2$$

where 1.34 is the hemoglobin oxygen content at 100% saturation (ml/g), Hb is the hemoglobin concentration (g/l) and $P_{(a-v)}O_2$ is the arterio-venous oxygen partial pressure difference (mmHg).

**Table 5.5.** Recommended flow rates (l/minute) for different surface areas and flow index

| Body surface area (m²) | Flow index 1.8 l/minute/m² | Flow index 2.2 l/minute/m² |
| --- | --- | --- |
| 1.60 | 2.88 | 3.52 |
| 1.80 | 3.24 | 3.96 |
| 2.00 | 3.60 | 4.40 |
| 2.20 | 3.96 | 4.84 |

Effective blood flow is that which actually results in maintenance of near-physiological tissue perfusion. Effective perfusion is reduced by anatomical shunting of arterial blood around the capillary bed to the venous circulation, e.g., via bronchial or pulmonary collaterals, and by the physiological shunt created by blood suctioned from the surgical field.

Indices of adequate total perfusion include pH, lactate and $S_vO_2$ (hemoglobin oxygen saturation in venous blood). A low $S_vO_2$ during CPB indicates an imbalance between $DO_2$ and $VO_2$ and requires a change in perfusion conditions. It can reflect insufficient pump flow, HCT, hemoglobin oxygen saturation, inadequate anesthesia or increasing temperature. All of these parameters should be optimized to ensure effective blood flow and consequent perfusion of organs.

In adults at normothermia, clinical and experimental data support a minimum flow index of 1.8 l/minute/m². Kirklin and Barratt-Boyes recommended a flow index of 2.2 l/minute/m² for adults at a temperature of 28°C or above. The patient's body surface area (m²) is worked out from a normogram plotting height in meters and weight in kilograms. Patients with a body surface area greater than 2 m² should have the flow maintained at 1.8–2.2 l/minute/m² to avoid excessively high flows through the machine leading to hemolysis.

Table 5.5 shows recommended flow rates for different surface areas.

Flow rates are reduced at lower body temperatures as $VO_2$ also decreases (see Appendix 5A).

## Hemodilution

As the CPB circuit is primed with crystalloid or colloid, hemodilution of the patient inevitably results. The degree of hemodilution caused by CPB can be calculated before initiating bypass so that the prime solution can be adjusted to incorporate packed red blood cells if unacceptable levels of anemia are anticipated.

$$CPB\ HCT = \frac{preop\ HCT \times PBV}{PBV + CPB\ prime\ volume}$$

where PBV = patient's blood volume (l) and CPB prime volume = extracorporal prime volume (l).

Benefits of hemodilution include reduced blood viscosity and an increase in microvascular blood flow, but these effects are partially counterbalanced by the reduction in oncotic pressure, which may promote tissue edema.

## Mean arterial blood pressure (MAP)

An acceptable MAP on CPB is that which provides adequate tissue perfusion. Adequate tissue perfusion is, however, also influenced by the pump flow rate and the core body temperature. MAP is determined by flow rate and arteriolar resistance. In general, higher pressures should be maintained in the presence of known cerebrovascular disease, in particular carotid stenosis, renal dysfunction, coronary disease or left ventricular hypertrophy.

On commencement of CPB there is a transient drop in systemic pressure. This is due to vasodilatation associated with the sudden decrease in blood viscosity resulting from hemodilution by the CPB prime solution and, secondarily, from the systemic inflammatory response (SIRS) associated with CPB. However, as CPB continues there is a gradual increase in perfusion pressure due to increasing vascular resistance. This is a result of equilibration of fluid between the vascular and tissue "compartments," hemoconcentration from diuresis, the increase in blood viscosity seen with hypothermia and the progressive increase in circulating levels of catecholamines and renin as part of the stress response to CPB.

It is important to emphasize that manipulation of MAP alone is not sufficient to guarantee adequate organ perfusion. Neither a low MAP with a high flow nor a high MAP with a low flow are sufficient in themselves. Whole body $DO_2$ must firstly be optimized and secondly, vascular resistance altered to bring the MAP into the autoregulatory range for critical organ beds, with due consideration to underlying pathophysiology.

## Pulmonary artery and left atrial pressure

On CPB the PA and LA pressures should be close to zero. PA or LA pressure monitoring is useful during CPB to assess left ventricular distension, in particular in cases where increase in blood flow back to the left heart is expected (cyanotic heart disease, large bronchial flow in chronic lung disease or aortic regurgitation). Care must be taken with PA catheters to ensure that migration of the catheter tip does not occur, leading to "wedging" and subsequent PA rupture or infarction of the lung.

## Central venous pressure

On CPB, CVP is expected to be close to zero and no more than in single digits. An increase in CVP indicates impaired venous drainage to the reservoir. The causes of an increase in CVP are inadequate cannula size, obstruction to the line or cannula tip and insufficient height difference between the patient and the reservoir to enable gravity siphon drainage. The consequence of an increase in CVP during bypass is to reduce effective perfusion of critical organs with resultant edema. The liver is particularly sensitive to reduced flow as nearly three-quarters of hepatic blood flow occurs at near venous pressure. If a persistently high CVP, uncorrected by attention to the factors mentioned above, is noted during CPB the patient's head and eyes should be closely observed for signs of engorgement and consideration given to altering the venous cannulation to improve drainage.

## Electrocardiogram

The ECG must be recorded throughout CPB to ensure that it remains isoelectric during cardioplegic arrest. Following removal of the aortic clamp and resumption of myocardial activity persistent ST segment changes may be related to ischemia resulting from inadequate re-vascularization, coronary ostial obstruction, e.g., by an incorrectly seated aortic valve prosthesis, or air/particulate embolization. Additionally, the ECG is useful in guiding the postoperative management of epicardial pacing.

## Temperature

The principal reason for hypothermic CPB is to protect the heart and other organs by reducing metabolic rate and thus oxygen requirements. In the myocardium, hypothermia sustains intracellular reserves of high-energy phosphates and preserves higher intracellular pH and electrochemical neutrality. Myocardial cooling can be achieved with cold cardioplegia, pouring cold topical solution on the heart and cooling jackets, as well as by systemic hypothermia. Systemic hypothermia is not uniform due to different blood flow to different vascular beds. High blood flow rates and slow cooling ensures less variation in systemic hypothermia. Temperature should be measured at multiple sites and the advantages and limitations of each site needs to be recognized. During cardiac surgery temperature can be measured in the following locations: nasopharynx, tympanic membrane, pulmonary artery, bladder or rectum, arterial inflow, water entering heat exchanger and venous return.

Nasopharyngeal temperature probes underestimate, but approximate to brain temperature, with the mixed venous temperature on the CPB circuit being an approximation of average body temperature. Bladder and rectal temperatures give an indication of core body temperatures, but these can be erroneous due to interference from varying urine production and fecal matter, respectively. These low blood flow sites tend to underestimate temperature so are particularly valuable following deeper levels of hypothermia. On re-warming the aim is to achieve uniform normothermia. To avoid rebound hypothermia after cessation of CPB, which occurs if too great a temperature gradient is allowed to develop between peripheral and core temperatures, vasodilators can be used to promote more uniform re-warming by distributing greater blood flow, and therefore heat, from the core to peripheries. The process of re-warming must be controlled to avoid rapid changes in temperature, or excessive blood temperatures, which can result in micro-bubble formation due to the reduced solubility of gases in blood as the temperature increases, denaturing of plasma proteins, hemolysis and cerebral injury. As a general guide for every 1°C drop in temperature there is an associated 7% drop in oxygen demand, i.e., a 7°C reduction in temperature results in a 50% drop in oxygen demand (see Table 5.6).

At less than <15°C oxygen is too tightly bound to hemoglobin and is therefore unavailable to tissues. In addition, the viscosity of the blood can be too high for effective flow through the CPB circuit.

## Urine volume

Urine volume on CPB is monitored as an indicator of renal perfusion. Indications for diuretic use during CPB include hyperkalemia, hemoglobinuria and hemodilution. Furosemide is used for treatment of hyperkalemia and mannitol is used to generate alkaline urine to treat hemoglobinuria.

## Transesophageal echocardiography (TOE)

TOE is applied increasingly as a routine part of surgery when intracardiac cavities are opened. It is a useful tool to assess adequacy of de-airing of the heart. In addition, TOE can be used to

**Table 5.6.** Hypothermia: temperature ranges and indications for use

| Hypothermia | Temperature (°C) | Use |
| --- | --- | --- |
| Tepid | 33–35 | Good for short operations, healthy patients with higher HCTs |
| Mild | 31–32 | Protection of beating heart and neurological systems |
| Moderate | 25–30 | Protection of non-beating heart and neurological systems |
| Deep | 15–20 | DHCA for typically 40–60 minutes |

assess intracardiac structures (valves, prostheses, septal walls, left and right ventricular out-flow tracts) and regional wall motility.

## Laboratory investigations

This is discussed in detail in Chapter 6.

Minimal monitoring during CPB requires measurement of $PO_2$, $PCO_2$, base excess, hemoglobin, HCT, pH, potassium, glucose and coagulation status using ACT.

## Termination of CPB

Table 5.7 provides a checklist of the basic conditions that need to be fulfilled before weaning can be attempted. Terminating CPB is a gradual process with constant communication between surgeon, anesthetist and perfusionist. The first step is for the perfusionist to restore the blood volume to the heart by gradual occlusion of the venous return. The patient is partially supported by the CPB machine with blood passing through both the heart and the lungs. The heart begins to eject blood when a critical volume is reached. The perfusionist continues to return blood from the venous reservoir to the patient whilst continuing to occlude the venous line until the patient is weaned from CPB. Termination of CPB is achieved by complete occlusion of the arterial and venous lines.

Transfusion of blood to the patient is still possible through the arterial cannula following cessation of CPB. The venous cannula is removed when the patient is stable and the process of reversing heparin with protamine is due to commence. Some surgeons leave the venous purse-string suture untied but snared to enable rapid re-insertion of a cannula for emergent return to CPB if required. Prior to protamine administration cardiotomy suction is stopped to avoid clotting within the bypass circuit. The protamine should be administered slowly due to its propensity for causing systemic vasodilatation and pulmonary vasoconstriction. Transfusion of residual blood from the pump is usually required to support cardiac filling during protamine administration; generally boluses of 100 ml are given, titrated against MAP and CVP, PA or LA pressures and direct observation of the heart. The aortic cannula is typically removed when protamine administration is completed, the patient is stable and there is no further requirement for transfusion of residual blood via the CPB machine. The two purse-string sutures on the aorta are tied to secure the cannulation site.

**Table 5.7.** Checklist before weaning from CPB

| |
|---|
| Patient position on operating table is neutral |
| Operation completed and vent sites closed |
| Hemostasis secured |
| Heart de-aired (confirmed with TOE if available) |
| Ventilation of lungs recommenced and adequate |
| Acceptable Hb/HCT, potassium, glucose, and acid–base status on arterial blood gas analysis |
| Acceptable core temperature achieved |
| Heart rhythm and rate appropriate |
| Parameters for initial filling pressure when off CPB are determined |
| Inotropic support prepared if necessary |

The remainder of the blood in the bypass circuit can be retained for transfusion by the anesthetist directly or it can be processed through a cell-salvage device to maximize the red cell concentration of this "pump blood." After transfusion a further dose of protamine may be administered to counteract the heparin in the pump blood.

Transition from CPB to physiological circulation is more often than not an uneventful process. In some circumstances, particularly when operating on patient's with severely impaired ventricular function, or if there has been a long ischemic period during the procedure, weaning from CPB may require measures to be taken to support the circulation. Such measures are discussed in Chapter 8.

# Appendix 5A: Protocol for the conduct of "routine" CPB

(Adapted, with permission, from London Perfusion Science Protocols.)

## 5A.1: Connection of the circuitry to the patient

- The surgeon will ask for the CPB lines to be divided
- The pump flow is slowly reduced and the venous line clamped, followed by the arterial line, beyond the recirculating Y-connector
- The surgeon will cannulate the aorta or peripheral arterial vessel
- If required, the arterial pump is continuously turned to assist an air free connection
- When the line is free of air the surgeon will connect the arterial line and confirm that the connection is satisfactory
- The clamp from the arterial line is removed and repositioned behind the recirculating Y-connector
- The swing on the "Tycos" gauge is checked
- If required, 50 ml blood is transfused to determine the adequacy of the swing
- Perfusionist should state there is a "good swing" if the gauge swings freely and reflects the patient's blood pressure
- If the perfusionist has any doubts about the cannulation, he must inform the surgeon immediately, continuing to voice his misgivings until he is confident that the cannula is satisfactorily placed
- Surgeon will cannulate the venous circulation (via RA, IVC and SVC or peripherally)
- Be prepared to use the pump suckers to deal with any blood loss
- Be prepared to transfuse the patient to replace this lost blood volume

## 5A.2: Initiating bypass

- If the gases have not yet been switched on, they are now correctly set according to the patient's rated flow
- The perfusionist must now clearly inform the medical staff that he/she is "going onto bypass"
- The clamp on the arterial line is removed and the pump is slowly turned at first, gradually increasing the rpm
- When going onto bypass with a centrifugal pump, forward pressure must be generated before the line clamp is removed. The drive motor is therefore turned on whilst the aortic line is still clamped, in order to generate sufficient forward pressure, to exceed the patient's arterial pressure; above 2000 rpm is usual

- The perfusionist must monitor the pressure on the line pressure (electronic or Tycos) during this stage, looking for any sign of obstruction: at the same time monitoring the venous and arterial pressures and, of course, monitoring the blood level in the venous reservoir, as the pump speed is increased
- Having raised the pressure on the venous side, the venous clamp is removed – more quickly if air has been left in the venous line – until this air has been removed. Perfusionists should then control the venous pressure with their clamp until they have achieved full rated flow for the patient
- The anesthetist should be informed when full flow has been achieved, so that ventilation may be discontinued
- Any difficulty in achieving a full venous return should be reported immediately to the surgeons, so that they may make any adjustment to the venous cannulation as may be necessary. Venous air should also be reported to the surgeon. It is important that an optimum venous return can be obtained at this stage
- The perfusionist must monitor the ECG at this stage, so that arrhythmias, particularly ventricular fibrillation (VF), may be noted early and action taken to prevent cardiac distension
- Once the aorta has been clamped, the required temperature has been achieved, cardioplegia has been administered, if required, and a steady state of perfusion has been attained, the first sample for blood gases, electrolytes, ACT, Hb/HCT and glucose is taken

## 5A.3: Patient flows

The flow required to meet a patient's metabolic requirements may need to be modified in certain circumstances (such as the presence of carotid disease). Using the patient's height and weight, the patient's surface area is obtained from a standard nomogram, and hence flows calculated for differing levels of metabolic requirement:

| Hypothermia | Temperature (°C) | Flow index (l/minute/m²) |
|---|---|---|
| Normothermia | 34–37 | 2.4 |
| Moderate hypothermia | 32–34 | 2.2 |
| Hypothermia | 28–32 | 1.8–2.0 |
| Profound hypothermia | <28 | 1.6 |

As a general rule, flows should be reduced with temperature (as metabolic requirement diminishes) and vice versa. Whilst individual cases may require special consideration, it is important to note the following:

Hypothermia is used as a technique in order that flows may be safely reduced. Too high a flow at a reduced temperature may:

- Cause blood damage
- Impede the surgery by flooding the field
- Cause an excessive rise in venous pressure
- Cause warming of the heart when cardioplegia has been used
- Cause underperfusion. Flows should correspond to temperature. Too low a flow during re-warming or at normothermia may lead to serious underperfusion

# 5A.4: The re-warming phase

The re-warming phase begins only after consultation with the surgeon. On re-warming, appropriate adjustments to gas flows and to blood flows must be made. This is a period during which a rapid drop in $S_vO_2$ may be experienced. A sample for all parameters should be taken during the mid-warming phase, in order to give sufficient time for any corrective action to be taken before coming off bypass. Final samples should be taken once a core temperature >35°C has been attained.

## 5A4.1: Re-warming

- The patient should be re-warmed using the arterial blood temperature and patient core temperature as guides to the rate and extent of re-warming
- The target arterial blood temperature is between 37.5 and 38°C. The upper limit should not be exceeded
- A gradient of 10°C between the water temperature in the heater–chiller unit and the arterial blood should not be exceeded
- Re-warming the patient to 37°C (nasopharyngeal) is usually a maximum, although surgeons vary in this regard
- Appropriate adjustments to gas flows and to blood flows must be made
- The rate of re-warming should be such as to allow time for distribution of heat between core and peripheral tissues, using vasodilators, if needed, to enhance peripheral blood flow and thus heat distribution
- Post-CPB an "after drop" in core temperature occurs as heat is redistributed from core to peripheral tissues; this after drop can be lessened if adequate time is allowed for thorough re-warming

## Suggested Further Reading

- Abel RM, Buckley MJ, Austen WG, Barnett GO, Beck CH Jr, Fischer JE. Etiology, incidence, and prognosis of renal failure following cardiac operations. Results of a prospective analysis of 500 consecutive patients. *J Thorac Cardiovasc Surg* 1976; **71**(3): 323–33.
- Bennett EV Jr, Fewel JG, Grover FL, Trinkle JK. Myocardial preservation: effect of venous drainage. *Ann Thorac Surg* 1983; **36**(2): 132–42.
- Hartman GS, Isom OW, Krieger KH. Retrograde autologous priming for cardiopulmonary bypass: a safe and effective means of decreasing hemodilution and transfusion requirements. *J Thorac Cardiovasc Surg* 1998; **115**(2): 426–39.
- Nuetzle, Bailey CP. New method for systemic arterial perfusion in extracorporeal circulation. *J Thorac Surg* 1959; **37**(6): 707–10 (no abstract available).
- Rosengart TK, DeBois W, O'Hara M, *et al.* Deairing of the venous drainage in standard extracorporeal circulation results in a profound reduction of arterial micro bubbles. *Thorac Cardiovasc Surg* 2006; **54**(1): 39–41.

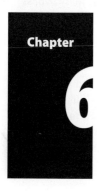

# Metabolic management during cardiopulmonary bypass

Kevin Collins and G. Burkhard Mackensen

The key to metabolic management during cardiopulmonary bypass (CPB) is the maintenance of adequate blood flow and oxygen delivery to the body's tissues. Utilizing the CPB machine, the perfusionist provides the optimum conditions necessary for operations on the heart, lungs or major vessels, while supporting the patient's physiological and metabolic needs.

> The perfect perfusion to me… is to be allowed to perform the necessary repair, however long that takes and yet leaving my patients looking like they've never been on bypass.
>
> Dr. Norman Shumway, Stanford University

## CPB-induced perturbations of patient metabolism and corrective interventions

CPB induces a unique set of physiological disturbances. The principal causes of metabolic derangement include:

- fluid priming of the CPB circuit;
- organ hypoperfusion; and
- changes in body temperature.

The causes, management and monitoring of metabolic parameters during CPB are discussed in this chapter.

## CPB primes, hemodilution, autologous priming and hemofiltration

### CPB circuit primes

All priming fluids cause hemodilution, which leads to a fall in the hematocrit (HCT), alterations in the volume of distribution of electrolytes and fluid shifts between the vascular and intercellular compartments. Every attempt should be made to minimize the volume of the CPB circuit. Use of small-diameter tubing and cannulae in the circuit, minimizing the length of circuit tubing, partially priming with autologous blood and using vacuum-assisted venous drainage all provide easy methods of reducing priming volume.

In the earliest days of cardiac surgery and CPB in the late 1950s, the prime was constituted to provide near normal HCT levels. However, with the advent of the use of hypothermia in the 1960s, intentional hemodilution became standard practice. Hemodilution is principally

*Cardiopulmonary Bypass,* ed. S. Ghosh, F. Falter and D. J. Cook. Published by Cambridge University Press.
© Cambridge University Press 2009.

**Table 6.1.** Expected HCT on CPB

| |
|---|
| HCT on CPB = red cell volume/system volume |
| Red cell volume = patient blood volume × pre-CPB HCT |
| System volume = patient blood volume + prime volume |
| Blood volume: |
| Adult – male: 70 ml/kg, female: 60 ml/kg |
| Child – 1–10 years: 80 ml/kg, 3–6 months: 85 ml/kg, 0–3 months: 90 ml/kg |

the result of the need for fluid priming of the CPB circuit, but also arises from the infusion of fluids during surgery and the administration of cardioplegia solution (CPS). Some degree of hemodilution is considered to be beneficial as:

- the reduction in blood viscosity minimizes CPB circuit sheer stresses upon blood, thereby lowering hemolysis rates; and
- reduced blood viscosity improves blood flow through capillary networks.

Utilizing weight-adjusted formulas, the desired HCT on CPB can be calculated as outlined in Table 6.1.

Further rationale for the use of hemodilution include reducing bank blood usage and the associated risks of transfusion, as well as respecting the wishes of patients not wanting to receive blood transfusions (e.g., Jehovah's Witness).

Hemodilution affects the concentration of plasma proteins. These colloids exert an oncotic pressure, holding water in the vascular compartment and so preventing the accumulation of water in interstitial spaces. Plasma proteins also bind a high proportion of drugs and electrolytes, maintaining a balance between their unbound, ionized state and their protein-bound state. Serum albumin (3.5–5.5 g/dl) constitutes 50–70% of the total protein with globulins (2–3.6 g/dl) comprising the bulk of the remainder.

Starches, modified animal colloids or human albumin may be added to CPB primes to increase their effective oncotic pressure. The composition of CPB primes is discussed in detail in Chapter 3.

## Autologous priming

Autologous priming (AP) utilizes the patient's blood to re-prime the CPB circuit upon initiation of CPB. Normal (antegrade) blood flow (Q) through the CPB circuit displaces the circuit prime with the patient's venous blood while diverting the crystalloid into a sterile bag. During the 10- to 20-second period required for AP, the patient is essentially being exsanguinated and the anesthetist must administer vasoconstrictors as required to maintain blood pressure. Alternatively, partial priming with autologous arterial blood can be achieved by retrograde drainage of 100–400 ml of blood via the arterial cannula into the cardiotomy reservoir. Depending on circuitry type, AP can significantly reduce the amount of crystalloid priming volume (e.g., from 1500–1800 ml to ~1100–1400 ml). AP can dramatically decrease the extent of hypotension, attributed to rapid hemodilution, commonly seen following the initiation of CPB. AP allows for higher HCT levels with slightly higher viscosities at warmer CPB temperatures (32–35°C) and still appears to avoid hemolysis from CPB circuit sheer stresses. AP also aids "normalization" of vascular oncotic pressures, thus decreasing fluid shifts and "third spacing."

**Table 6.2.** Hemodynamic calculations for CPB

| |
|---|
| BSA = √ (kg × cm/3600) |
| CPB flow (Q) = CI × BSA |
| CI = CO/BSA |
| SVR = (MAP – CVP/CO) × 80 |

BSA – body surface area; CI – cardiac index; CO – cardiac output; CPB – cardiopulmonary bypass; CVP – central venous pressure; Q – blood flow; SVR – systemic vascular resistance; MAP – mean arterial pressure.

**Table 6.3.** $O_2$ calculations for CPB

| |
|---|
| $VO_2 = (S_aO_2 - S_vO_2)$ (1.34) (Hb) + $(P_aO_2 - P_vO_2)$ (0.003) |
| $O_2$ capacity = (1.34) (Hb) + (0.003) $(PO_2)$ |
| $O_2$ content = (1.34) (Hb) $(S_aO_2$ or $S_vO_2)$ + (0.003) $(PO_2)$ |
| CPB $O_2$ consumption = $(aO_2 - vO_2)$ (Q l/minute) (10) |
| CPB $O_2$ transfer = $[(S_aO_2 - S_vO_2)$ (1.34) (Hb) (Q ml/minute)] /100 |

$aO_2$ content – arterial oxygen content ; CPB – cardiopulmonary bypass; Hb – hemoglobin; $P_aO_2$ – oxygen arterial partial pressure; $P_vO_2$ - oxygen venous partial pressure; Q – blood flow; $S_aO_2$ – arterial oxygen saturation; $S_vO_2$ – mixed venous oxygen saturation; $vO_2$ content – venous oxygen content.

# CPB flow rates

The perfusionist calculates a CPB blood flow (Q) utilizing the patient's body surface area (BSA) and cardiac index (CI) (see Table 6.2). Insufficient flow can result in inadequate tissue perfusion. Metabolic acidosis during CPB is almost always the result of hypoperfusion leading to oxygen delivery inadequate to meet metabolic demands for aerobic respiration. Oxygen consumption ($VO_2$) is thus a major determinant of CPB flow requirements (see Table 6.3).

## Hypoperfusion

CPB-related hypoperfusion may be intentional or unintentional. The most common intentional causes of transient periods of hypoperfusion are induced by the cardiac surgeon. Manipulation of the heart may impede venous blood return to the CPB circuit necessitating a reduction in flow. Frequently, the surgeon requests the perfusionist to reduce flow to permit safe application or removal of the aortic cross-clamp, decrease surgical bleeding or to empty and decompress the heart.

Reduction of pump flow, for unintentional reasons, is nearly always caused by poor venous return to the circuit, usually due to a venous cannula that has been advanced too far or surgical distortion of the vena cavae and heart, although improper arterial cannulation, movement of the cannulae after placement or an incorrectly occluded arterial roller pump head sometimes may occur.

# Temperature and hypothermia

The temperature of the patient whilst on CPB is one of the most profound determinants of the requirements for perfusion. Systemic $O_2$ consumption, $VO_2$, is reduced by approximately 50% for every 7°C reduction in core temperature below normothermia (30°C = 50%, 23°C = 25%, 16°C = 12.5% metabolic demand of the same organ at 37°C; see table 6.4). As such, relatively

**Table 6.4.** Classification of hypothermia

Mild: 36–34°C

Moderate: 33–28°C

Severe: 27–22°C

Deep: <21°C

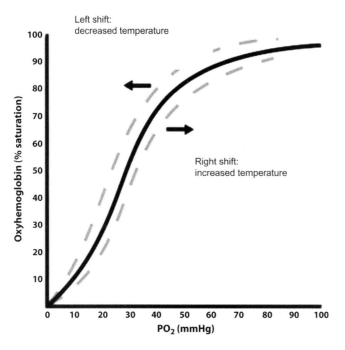

**Figure 6.1** Oxyhemoglobin dissociation curve.

small decreases in temperature markedly reduce the requirements for systemic $O_2$ delivery, making moderate reductions in pump flow or HCT tolerable, such that $DO_2$ remains sufficient to meet $VO_2$.

Left and right shifts in the oxygen–hemoglobin dissociation curve also occur with temperature changes during CPB (see Figure 6.1). At lower temperatures hemoglobin has a greater affinity for binding oxygen, consequently oxygen is also released less readily and the dissociation curve is shifted to the left. At higher temperatures the converse is true and the curve is shifted to the right.

Pump flow rate must be adjusted with due consideration to temperature if the metabolic demands for oxygen are to be matched by delivery. Typical flow rates over a range of temperatures are shown in the Appendix 5A.

# Deep hypothermic circulatory arrest (DHCA)

Deep hypothermic circulatory arrest is discussed in detail in Chapter 10, but is briefly mentioned here for completeness. Certain cardiac procedures require DHCA, rather than just conventional mild to moderate hypothermia, usually because the aorta cannot be cross-clamped or total absence of blood flow is required to enable surgical access. DHCA is used to dramatically lower the body's metabolic demand while protecting organs, particularly the brain, during a period in which perfusion is suspended. This technique utilizes profound hypothermia, with or without the use of aortic cross-clamping and delivery of cardioplegia, to facilitate surgery to the left ventricular outflow tract, aortic valve, ascending aorta or great vessels. Pediatric palliative and corrective surgical procedures also frequently necessitate periods of DHCA. Procedurally dictated, intermittent "low-flow" (5–15 ml/kg/minute) states may be employed during DHCA to deliver oxygenated blood to the brain via antegrade (ACP) and retrograde cerebral perfusion (RCP). During ACP in adult patients, mean arterial pressure (MAP) should be ≤65 mmHg, and during RCP the central venous pressure (CVP) should be ≤25 mmHg.

# pH, acid–base, blood gases and electrolytes

## pH and acid–base

The normal pH of arterial blood is 7.4 (± 0.05). Bicarbonate and non-bicarbonate systems play important roles in buffering pH changes.

### Bicarbonate system

The bicarbonate buffer system (carbonic acid $H_2CO_3$ and bicarbonate $HCO_3^-$) is considered to be the most important mechanism for physiological regulation of pH. It possesses approximately 53% of the total buffering capacity of body fluids. Exogenous sodium bicarbonate is easily administered during CPB. It should be noted that bicarbonate's molecular weight is small enough to allow its passage across the semipermeable fibers of the hemofilter and may thus be removed with the effluent product or "plasma water waste" if hemofiltration is used during CPB. The simple formula [(body weight (kg) × 0.3)/2] × base deficit = mmol $NaHCO_3^-$ needed to yield base excess equal to 0 is often used when treating persistent acidosis.

### Non-bicarbonate buffers

- **Inorganic phosphate buffers** are important in regulating pH in the intracellular and renal tubular fluids. Inorganic phosphates, like bicarbonate, are removed during hemofiltration.
- **Plasma proteins** possess significant buffering capacity because of the ionic nature of their amino acid structure and because of their high plasma concentrations. Plasma proteins are not removed during hemofiltration because of their larger molecular size.
- **Hemoglobin and oxyhemoglobin** play a major role in buffering hydrogen ions at the tissue level. Considered the most important of the non-bicarbonate pH buffers, hemoglobin is not removed during hemofiltration because of the size of the red blood cell.

### Metabolic acidosis and alkalosis

Metabolic acidosis is usually due to systemic $O_2$ delivery ($DO_2$) during bypass not meeting systemic $O_2$ demand ($VO_2$). The options to address this are to increase pump flow or HCT, thereby increasing $DO_2$, or to reduce $VO_2$ by decreasing temperature or possibly by increasing depth of anesthesia. Failing this, administration of sodium bicarbonate, or the use of hemofiltration (ultrafiltration) may correct the acidosis.

CPB-related metabolic alkalosis is usually due to a reduction in serum potassium levels (e.g., due to increased urine output or hemofiltration) and is best treated by titrated administration of potassium chloride.

### Respiratory acidosis and alkalosis

Respiratory acidosis is the result of insufficient removal of $CO_2$ from the patient's blood by the membrane oxygenator. Increasing the sweep gas rate through the membrane oxygenator will facilitate the transfer or elimination of excess $CO_2$ from the patient's blood. Conversely, respiratory alkalosis is the result of excessive $CO_2$ removal.

# Alpha-stat and pH-stat strategies for blood gas management

The optimal pH management strategy during hypothermic cardiopulmonary bypass is as yet undetermined. The two main strategies utilized clinically, alpha-stat and pH-stat, differ in their approach to the acid–base alterations that occur with hypothermia. As blood temperature falls, gas solubility rises and the partial pressure of carbon dioxide decreases ($PCO_2$ decreases 4.4% for every °C drop in temperature). With alpha-stat management, arterial gas samples are not corrected for sample temperature and the resulting alkalosis remains untreated during cooling; with pH-stat management, arterial blood gas samples are temperature corrected and carbon dioxide is added to the gas inflow of the CPB circuit so that the $PCO_2$, and hence pH, is corrected to the same levels as during normothermia. The advocates of alpha-stat point to potential benefits in terms of the function of intracellular enzyme systems and the advantage of preserving cerebral autoregulation. Proponents of pH-stat, which results in cerebral vasodilation, cite as advantages higher levels of oxygen delivery to the brain and enhanced distribution of blood flow. However, the higher cerebral blood flows associated with pH-stat also have the potential to carry more gaseous or particulate emboli to the brain.

Alpha-stat management is based on the concept that the dissociation constant, pK, of the histidine imidazole group changes with temperature in a manner nearly identical to physiological blood buffers. Hence, the ionization state ($\alpha$) of this group stays the same, irrespective of temperature. As the imidazole group's ionization state is a key determinant of intracellular protein function, advocates of alpha-stat management contend that this strategy promotes normal protein charge states and function, even at low temperatures.

The pH-stat approach increases the total carbon dioxide content of the blood as the temperature falls in order to maintain fixed temperature-corrected pH values. The optimal pH of most enzymatic reactions does vary with hypothermia, mostly in accordance with the predictions of the alpha-stat hypothesis. Hence, the relative acidosis of pH-stat would be expected to lower enzymatic reaction rates. Whether this is beneficial in reducing energy consumption, or harmful by impairing key cellular homeostatic mechanisms, is unclear.

Differences in alpha-stat and pH-stat management become progressively greater as temperature is reduced so the effect is quite profound below 25°C, but above 32°C, quantitatively, the change in $CO_2$ solubility is small and of much less clinical and physiological relevance. This is further evident when one appreciates how little CPB time most adult cardiac surgical patients spend at hypothermic temperatures. Most cases are conducted with mild hypothermia and in those much of CPB time is spent transitioning to, or from, those temperatures; the actual time on CPB spent below 32°C may only be 25% of the total CPB time. Thus, although frequently discussed, alpha-stat versus pH-stat management is of little actual relevance in most adult cardiac surgery.

# Electrolytes

## Potassium (K$^+$)

Hyperkalemia is the most common electrolyte disturbance during CPB. Potassium levels can be lowered using diuretics, insulin and dextrose administration, or hemofiltration. The treatment of choice is dictated by the potassium level, the persistence of rise in potassium levels and the presence or absence of electrophysiological disturbances. Serum potassium levels transiently rise with the administration of cardioplegia and this will usually correct without treatment within a short period after ceasing delivery of cardioplegia. Potassium levels in the range 5.5–6.5 mmol/l can be treated with administration of a diuretic, usually furosemide 20–40 mg. In some centers, levels between 6.5 and 7 mmol/l are treated using insulin and dextrose infusions. Levels above 7 mmol/l or persistently raised potassium levels can be lowered using "zero balance hemofiltration." A crystalloid solution, typically normal saline, is added to the CPB circuit to maintain circulatory volume and then removed by hemofiltration causing concomitant removal of potassium. As this technique can result in the loss of significant amounts of bicarbonate through the hemofilter, it should be replaced using sodium bicarbonate titrated to blood bicarbonate levels.

The urgency or need to treat hyperkalemia should in part be determined by the presence or absence of electrophysiological disturbance. In the absence of ECG changes, moderate hyperkalemia may not require treatment. If treatment is chosen, its effect should not be longer than the anticipated period of hyperkalemia. It is important to note that during CPB extracellular potassium may rise but typically, even untreated, increases in K$^+$ levels are nearly always transient, as the extracellular potassium concentration in the plasma is quite small relative to the intracellular capacity for its uptake. Rapid shifts to the intracellular space and urinary excretion often correct K$^+$ levels quite quickly after CPB.

Hypokalemia, usually less than 4.5 mmol/l, is treated by administration of potassium chloride, normally in 10–20 mmol boluses. It is worth bearing in mind that rapid bolus administration of potassium during CPB may cause transient vasodilatation. Potassium levels alter with temperature. Treatment should be undertaken in the context of:

- temperature;
- the rate of rise of the potassium level;
- the persistence of that level; and
- the point during surgery at which it is occurring.

Ideally, potassium is finally corrected before separation from CPB using results of electrolyte measurements taken at a body temperature of not less than 35°C.

## Calcium (Ca$^{2+}$)

Calcium levels are reduced by hemodilution, chelation by preservatives in bank blood or by hemofiltration. Low serum Ca$^{2+}$ levels are generally corrected close to the termination of CPB, when the aortic cross-clamp has been removed, a cardiac rhythm has been established and the temperature is approaching normothermia. One gram (or 3–5 mg/kg) of calcium chloride is usually all that is required to normalize serum ionized calcium levels (1–1.5 mmol/l). Administration of Ca$^{2+}$ may exacerbate reperfusion injury and should be avoided immediately before or after cross-clamp removal. Timing of administration can be guided by normalization of cardiac conduction indicating adequate reperfusion.

## Magnesium (Mg$^+$)

Magnesium depletion occurs during CPB if hemofiltration is used or if there is high volume diuresis, particularly with loop diuretics. In these situations, a 2 mg bolus of Mg$^+$ may be added empirically into the circuit after the core temperature has reached 34°C and the aortic cross-clamp has been removed. Ideally, if Mg$^+$ levels are available, Mg$^+$ administration should be titrated according to blood levels.

## Phosphate

Phosphate levels are commonly low after major cardiac surgery. This frequently occurs in the immediate postoperative period and is associated with significant respiratory and cardiac morbidity. Therefore, phosphate levels should be routinely measured after surgery, especially in patients with a complicated or prolonged intraoperative course, so that appropriate replacement therapy may be started in a timely manner.

## Glucose

Phosphate levels on CPB tend to increase as a result of the physiological stress response to major surgery. Values may exceed 20 mmol/l in diabetic patients without treatment. Non-diabetic patients' serum glucose levels can also rise; levels of 10–15 mmol/l are not uncommon. Continuous insulin infusions of 5–15 U/hour may be required during CPB. Hyperglycemia is associated with poor patient outcomes. Specifically, perioperative hyperglycemia has been associated with higher incidences of mediastinitis, wound infections and neurocognitive deficits. Conflicting literature regarding both the ideal and acceptable intraoperative and postoperative glucose levels exists. However, recent studies have shown mixed results from attempts at aggressive management of CPB-related hyperglycemia. The results range from favorable outcomes, to little or no association between reducing serum glucose levels and reduction in postoperative complications, to adverse patient outcomes associated with the tight control of CPB-related hyperglycemia. It is generally believed that normal (4.0–5.5 mmol/l) serum glucose levels during CPB are ultimately desirable. Consistent achievement of this goal remains elusive at this time. Postoperative hypoglycemia, equally as dangerous and undesirable as hyperglycemia, can result from clinicians "overshooting" in their attempts at serum glucose reduction.

## Lactate

Lactate is a major end product of glucose metabolism and gives an indication of the metabolic status during CPB. Most patients exhibit a progressive increase in plasma lactate during CPB. Lactate levels increase two- to threefold during normothermic and hypothermic CPB. During periods of hypoperfusion or decreased liver function, usually secondary to hypothermia, serum lactate levels can increase even further (four- to eightfold). Re-warming the patient and increasing flow rates usually helps to lower lactate levels.

## Hemofiltration (Ultrafiltration)

This allows selective separation of plasma water and low-molecular-weight solutes from the blood's cellular and plasma protein. Hemofilter membranes are composed of thousands of semipermeable hollow fibers (polysulfone, polyacrylonitrile or cellulose acetate fibers), each with an internal diameter of ~200 μm. Hollow fiber pore size determines which plasma solutes will be removed. Pore size usually ranges between 10 and 35 angstroms, removing molecules $\leq 20\,000$ Daltons. The sieving coefficient is a measure of hemofilter efficiency and is directly related to solute molecular size. Solutes with weights $\leq 11\,000$ Daltons ($Na^+$, $K^+$, $Ca^{2+}$, $Mg^+$, urea, creatinine, chloride, phosphorous, $HCO_3^-$, C3a, C5a, IL-1, IL-6, TNF-$\alpha$) have a sieving coefficient of 1, indicating they are filtered at the same concentration as they exist in the blood. Larger molecules $>20\,000$ Daltons (hemoglobin, globulin, fibrinogen, blood cells, platelets, albumin and clotting factors) are unable to pass through the hemofilter fiber pores. The hydrostatic pressure differential, or transmembrane pressure (TMP), across the hemofilter rather than the osmotic pressures, as in hemodialysis, creates the separation of solutes and fluids. Application of vacuum to the effluent side of the hemofilter will improve solute and fluid filtration rates (up to 180 ml/minute). TMP (100–500 mmHg) is the mean of the hemofilter inlet (PI) and outlet (PO) pressures plus vacuum (PV): TMP=PI + PO/2 + PV. The combination of these pressures determines the filtration rate.

## Drug dilution and loss

The CPB circuit adds as much as 1800 ml to the adult patient's circulating volume, especially in institutions that do not employ prime-reducing techniques (AP, vacuum-assisted venous drainage and microcircuitry).

Institution of CPB results in an immediate dilution of drug concentrations. A new equilibrium between protein-bound and free ionized drug concentrations is established. Drug clearance and the intensity of biological effect are proportional to the concentration of free (unbound) drug, thus the pharmacodynamic effects of drugs are not necessarily altered if the concentration of free drug is maintained.

The effect of CPB on drug concentrations is complex and also influenced by a number of factors such as temperature and the type of materials used in the CPB circuit; certain types of plastics and coatings on oxygenator membranes are more prone to binding drugs than others.

## Monitoring of patient metabolic and physiological parameters

### Arterial and venous blood gases and electrolytes

In-line real-time blood gas analysis has become the "gold standard" for extracorporeal perfusion. These arterial and venous analyzers utilize disposable sensors that attach directly to the arterial and venous lines of the CPB circuit, providing a luminal surface interface for blood leaving the oxygenator and for blood returning from the patient. Arterial sensors provide pH, $PO_2$, $PCO_2$, BE, $HCO_3^-$ and $S_aO_2$ data. The venous sensor generally provides HCT, hemoglobin and mixed venous oxygen saturation ($S_vO_2$) measurements. Some in-line devices will also provide a continuous calculation of oxygen consumption based on pump flow and the arterio-venous oxygen differential.

If in-line blood gas monitoring is not available, intermittent samples should be taken at 30-minute intervals for analysis. Most blood gas machines provide data on blood gases, acid–base status, hematocrit, hemoglobin, electrolytes and glucose.

### $S_vO_2$

During CPB $S_vO_2$ is an indicator of the matching of $DO_2$ and $VO_2$. As the margin between systemic $O_2$ delivery and demand narrows, $O_2$ extraction increases and $S_vO_2$ is reduced.

Reduced depth of anesthesia or degree of muscular paralysis by muscle relaxant drugs, low inspired oxygen concentration in the fresh gas flow mixture or anemia all decrease $S_vO_2$. However, if these parameters have been optimized, low $S_vO_2$ values generally indicate hypoperfusion and should prompt an increase in pump flow rate to improve oxygen delivery. If the ability to increase flow is limited by venous return, then increasing $DO_2$ by increasing HCT, or reducing $VO_2$ by reducing temperature, is indicated. However, the $S_vO_2$ value should always also be interpreted in the context of core temperature. The solubility and hemoglobin binding affinity of oxygen increases with hypothermia, whilst organ metabolic demand decreases, resulting in increased $S_vO_2$ if perfusion is adequate. Venous saturations of 65–75% are typical at temperatures of 37–35°C, 76–85% at temperatures of 34–32°C, and 85–100% at temperatures of 32–16°C.

## Suggested Further Reading

- Butterworth J, Wagenknecht LE, Legault C, *et al*. Attempted control of hyperglycemia during cardiopulmonary bypass fails to improve neurologic or neurobehavioral outcomes in patients without diabetes mellitus undergoing coronary artery bypass grafting. *J Thorac Cardiovasc Surg* 2005; **130**: 1319.

- Gandhi GY, Nuttall GA, Abel MD, *et al*. Intensive intraoperative insulin therapy versus conventional glucose management during cardiac surgery: a randomized trial. *Ann Intern Med* 2007; **146**: 233–43.

- Gravlee GP, Davis RF, Stammers AH, Ungerleider R, eds. *Cardiopulmonary Bypass: Principles and Practice*, 3rd ed. Philadelphia: Wolters Kluwer Health/ Lippincott Williams & Wilkins; 2008.

- Grigore AM, Grocott HP, Mathew JP, *et al*. The rewarming rate and increased peak temperature alter neurocognitive outcome after cardiac surgery. *Anesth Analg* 2002; **94**: 4–10.

- Grocott HP, Mackensen GB, Grigore AM, *et al*. Postoperative hyperthermia is associated with cognitive dysfunction after coronary artery bypass graft surgery. *Stroke* 2002; **33**: 537–41.

- Mackensen GB, Grocott HP, Newman MF. Cardiopulmonary bypass and the brain. In Kay PH, Munsch CM, eds. *Techniques in Extracorporeal Circulation*, 4th ed. London: Oxford University Press; 2004: 148–76.

- McAlister FA, Man J, Bistritz L, *et al*. Diabetes and coronary artery bypass surgery: an examination of perioperative glycemic control and outcomes. *Diabetes Care* 2003; **26**: 1518–24.

- Puskas F, Grocott H, White W, *et al*. Intraoperative hyperglycemia and cognitive decline after CABG. *Ann Thorac Surg* 2007; **84**: 1467–73.

- Reed CC, Stafford TB. *Cardiopulmonary Bypass*, 2nd ed. Houston: Texas Medical Press; 1985.

- Watkins, JG. *Arterial Blood Gases: A Self-Study Manual*. Philadelphia: Lippincott Williams and Wilkins; 1985.

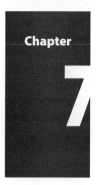

# Myocardial protection and cardioplegia

Constantine Athanasuleas and Gerald D. Buckberg

Optimal outcomes after cardiac surgery are dependent on several factors; primarily these are appropriate patient selection, precise surgical technique and intraoperative protection of viable myocardium. Myocardial damage may be associated with cardiopulmonary bypass (CPB) to varying degrees and influences morbidity and mortality. Cardioplegia, the solution used to protect the myocardium intraoperatively, in the period during which the heart is isolated from the circulation and hence ischemic, may differ in composition, route of administration and method of delivery to the heart. This chapter reviews the rationale for the use of cardioplegia, techniques of administration, components of different cardioplegia solutions and applications of cardioplegia in different surgical interventions.

## Myocardial damage during cardiopulmonary bypass

Damage to the myocardium can occur during short or long operations, but is more likely under certain clinical circumstances. These include prolonged aortic cross-clamp times, impaired ventricular function, concomitant valve or aortic surgery with coronary bypass, re-operation and operation during acute coronary ischemia.

During CPB, the aorta is usually clamped to provide a dry operative field with good visibility. If the heart continues to beat during aortic cross-clamping, intracellular depletion of high-energy phosphates ensues and results in impaired recovery of function. Intermittent cross-clamping with multiple periods of reperfusion has been shown to be suboptimal because episodes of reperfusion injury may occur following each release of the aortic clamp. The technique of cross-clamp and fibrillation, as an alternative method to using cardioplegia to provide a bloodless field and non-beating heart, engenders multiple short periods of ischemia followed by reperfusion. This may further potentiate, rather than prevent, ischemic damage, as redistribution of flow away from the vulnerable subendocardial muscle occurs.

Postoperatively, myocardial damage can be detected by electrocardiography, echocardiography, radioactive imaging studies and cardiac magnetic resonance imaging. Chemical markers of damage include troponin or creatine phosphokinase release. The clinical manifestations of myocardial damage may present as low cardiac output syndrome due to impaired myocardial contractility, dysrhythmias, decreased ventricular compliance or segmental myocardial wall motion abnormalities.

## Goals and principles of myocardial protection

The goal of myocardial protection with cardioplegia is to prevent myocardial injury during the periods of intentional ischemia that are required to perform cardiac operations. This can be accomplished by adjusting myocardial metabolic requirements both during the phase of no perfusion, and following reperfusion, in such a way as to minimize the deleterious effects of prolonged ischemia.

*Cardiopulmonary Bypass,* ed. S. Ghosh, F. Falter and D. J. Cook. Published by Cambridge University Press.
© Cambridge University Press 2009.

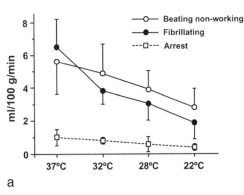 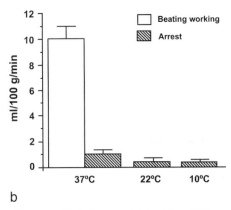

a          b

**Figure 7.1** (a) Left ventricular oxygen requirements of the beating, empty, fibrillating, arrested heart from 37°C to 22°C. Note the lowest requirements during arrest. (b) The left ventricular oxygen requirements of a beating/working heart and an arrested heart at 37°C, 22°C and 10°C.

The principal determinants of myocardial energy utilization are left ventricular end-diastolic wall tension (LVEDP) and electromechanical activity; limitation of both of these parameters can thus limit myocardial metabolic demand.

During diastole, with low LVEDP, myocardial oxygen consumption and energy substrate utilization is minimized. The rapid attainment of diastolic cardiac arrest at the onset of the ischemic period following application of the aortic cross-clamp effectively places the heart in a state of hibernation, particularly if the myocardium is simultaneously cooled.

Electromechanical activity raises oxygen demand during ischemia. Therefore, ideally, all electrical activity must cease during cardioplegia-induced cardiac arrest. Hypothermia, which in itself lowers basal metabolic rate and thus helps to reduce myocardial electrical activity, was used in thousands of operations in the early years of cardiac surgery. Topical cold saline or iced slush was poured over the heart into the pericardial cavity after aortic cross-clamping. Though effective for shorter periods of cross-clamping, this method becomes limiting following ischemic periods exceeding 1 hour. Subsequently, infusion of cold cardioplegia solutions into the myocardium to rapidly stop electromechanical activity and simultaneously reduce temperature in all myocardial layers has become the preferred method of cooling the heart (see Figure 7.1).

Interventions that maximize high-energy phosphate production, while minimizing high-energy phosphate utilization and intracellular calcium accumulation during ischemia and reperfusion, are effective in delaying or preventing the onset of ischemic necrosis and in aiding recovery of function following reperfusion. Examples of methods to maximize high-energy phosphate production include preoperative glucose and glycogen loading, intraoperative infusions of glucose, insulin and potassium, or the addition of Kreb's cycle intermediates, glutamate and aspartate, to cardioplegic solutions.

## Components of cardioplegia

The constitution of cardioplegia solutions varies according to individual surgeons and institutional preferences. The composition of cardioplegic solutions has been described as being similar to either the ionic composition of extracellular or of intracellular fluid depending on the content of sodium, potassium, calcium and magnesium of a given type of cardioplegia. Cardioplegia solutions can be further categorized according to whether they are crystalloid or blood based. The essential requirement for attainment of rapid diastolic cardiac arrest, however, renders potassium (20–40 mEq/l), which causes membrane depolarization, an essential ingredient of all cardioplegia solutions.

Other components common to cardioplegia solutions include sodium (100–200 mEq/l) and chloride ions. Sodium minimizes the transcellular sodium gradient and so reduces intracellular edema; marked extracellular hyponatremia (<50 mEql), together with excessive potassium-induced membrane depolarisation, alters the $Na^+/Ca^{2+}$ exchange mechanisms in such a way as to promote intracellular $Ca^{2+}$ accumulation causing damage to sarcolemma membranes. Chloride ions maintain the electroneutrality of the solution.

Modification of cardioplegia to produce a solution that provides optimal preservation of myocardial function has led to a variety of additions to the "basic" ingredients, for example one of the most established blood cardioplegia preparations contains citrate phosphate dextrose (CPD), to limit calcium influx during ischemia, and tromethamine (tris-hydroxymethyl aminomethane, THAM), a buffer that prevents acidosis. THAM diffuses into the intravascular space, "captures" the $CO_2$ produced by metabolic acidosis and improves myocardial performance.

The original cardioplegic solutions used for many years consisted of crystalloid solutions with various additives. The most widely used is the St. Thomas' Hospital solution. Calcium, in low concentration, is included in the solution to ensure that there is no likelihood of calcium paradox during reperfusion and to maintain integrity of cell membranes. Magnesium may help stabilize the myocardial membrane by inhibiting a myosin phosphorylase, which protects ATP reserves for postischemic activity. The protective effects of magnesium and potassium have been shown to be additive. Procaine, a local anesthetic, is included in low concentration, to counteract the vasocontrictive effects of particulate contaminants in the infusion and so promote even distribution.

St. Thomas' solution is usually buffered by the addition of sodium bicarbonate just prior to use; this renders the solution slightly alkaline and helps compensate for the metabolic acidosis that accompanies ischemia. Commercially prepared bags of ready diluted St. Thomas' cardioplegia are available as an alternative to diluting the concentrate with Ringer's, but differ slightly from the original St Thomas' preparation.

Hypothermic crystalloid cardioplegia has certain disadvantages, including the fact that it inhibits the enzyme $Na^+/K^+$ adenosine triphosphatase, which is intrinsic to the function of transmembrane ion pumps, thereby producing myocardial edema and consequent activation of platelets, leukocytes and complement.

Blood cardioplegia largely replaced crystalloid cardioplegia in most centers several years ago. It consists of four parts of blood to one part crystalloid cardioplegia solution. This limits the systemic hemodilution seen with crystalloid cardioplegia during repeated infusions. Blood cardioplegia maintains oncotic pressure, is a natural buffering agent, has advantageous rheological properties and is a free radical scavenger. It also limits reperfusion injury in the acutely ischemic myocardium. Experimental studies have shown that normal hearts subjected to up to 4 hours of ischemia have complete recovery of function when intermittent cold blood cardioplegia is infused. Cold blood cardioplegia alone, however, does not totally avoid injury. The Kreb's cycle amino acids glutamate and aspartate are depleted during episodes of intermittent blood cardioplegia administration. They are especially depleted in chronically ischemic hearts and may be replenished by using blood cardioplegia with added glutamate and aspartate, often referred to as "substrate-enhanced cardioplegia." Blood cardioplegia, with or without substrate enhancement, may be infused as a warm solution to optimize the

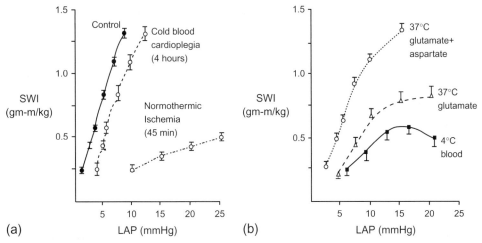

**Figure 7.2** (a) Left ventricular function in normal hearts subjected to 4 hours of aortic clamping with blood cardioplegia every 20 minutes compared with depressed function after 45 minutes of normothermic arrest without cardioplegia. (b) Left ventricular function when jeopardized hearts undergoing 45 minutes of normothermic ischemia are subjected to 2 more hours of aortic clamping. Note (1) no further improvement when only cold cardioplegic perfusate is given over the 45 minute arrest period, (2) progressively increased recovery when the cardioplegic solution is supplemented with warm glutamate and aspartate during induction of cardioplegia and reperfusion with intermittent cold doses of blood every 20 minutes of supplemental aortic clamping. LAP = left atrial pressure; SWI = stroke work index.

**Table 7.1.** Composition of crystalloid (STH1) and blood-based St. Thomas' Hospital cardioplegic (BSTH1) solutions (concentrations delivered to heart)

| Ionic composition | STH1 | BSTH1 |
|---|---|---|
| $Na^+$ (mmol/l) | 144 | 142 |
| $K^+$ (mmol/l) | 20 | 20 |
| $Mg^{2+}$ (mmol/l) | 16 | 16 |
| $Ca^{2+}$ (mmol/l) | 2.2 | 1.7 |
| $HCO_3^-$ (mmol/l) | 0* | 30–40 |
| Procaine (mmol/l) | 1 | 1 |
| pH | 5.5–7.0 | 7.4 |
| Hematocrit | 0 | 10–12% |
| Osmolarity (mOsmol/kg $H_2O$) | 300–320 | 310–330 |

Note: * $NaHCO_3$ added prior to use, increasing $HCO_3^-$ and pH.
Note: These are high $K^+$ solutions; low $K^+$ solutions (10 mmol/l) may be used for additional doses.

metabolic rate of repair, just prior to removal of the aortic cross-clamp, at the end of the intended ischemic period. This warm phase has been referred to as the "hot shot" of cardioplegia. It enhances cellular assimilation of the substrates (see Figure 7.2), augmenting the rate of recovery of myocardial contractility. Some surgeons also infuse a small volume of warm blood cardioplegia followed by cold cardioplegia to induce cardiac arrest at the commencement of the ischemic period, on the basis that this "feeds" the heart, i.e., provides a more physiological delivery of oxygen and substrates for the period of ischemia.

**Table 7.2.** Substrate-enhanced blood cardioplegia solution (high K⁺)

| Additive | Concentration delivered* |
|---|---|
| K⁺ (2 mEq/ml) | 16–20 mmol/l |
| THAM (0.3 mol/l) | pH 7.5–7.7 |
| Citrate–phosphate–dextrose | 0.2–0.4 mmol/l |
| Aspartate | 13 mmol/l |
| Glutamate | 13 mmol/l |
| Dextrose 50% | <400 mg/l |
| Dextrose 5% | 380–400 mOsm |

* When mixed with blood in a 4:1 ratio.

**Table 7.3.** "Multi-dose" low-potassium cold blood cardioplegia solution

| Additive | Concentration delivered* |
|---|---|
| K⁺ (2 mEq/ml) | 8–10 mmol/l |
| THAM (0.3 mol/l) | pH 7.6–7.8 |
| Citrate–phosphate–dextrose | 0.5–0.6 mmol/l |
| Dextrose 5% | 380–400 mOsm |

* When mixed with blood in a 4:1 ratio.

Compositions of typical crystalloid and blood cardioplegia solutions are shown in Tables 7.1, 7.2 and 7.3.

# Cardioplegia delivery

Cardioplegia delivery systems generally comprise an infusion system with in-line pressure monitors, a cardioplegic heat exchanger for cold and warm perfusion, and cannulae for antegrade and retrograde delivery. For further details about cannulae and cardioplegia delivery please see Chapter 1.

# Routes of cardioplegia delivery

To be effective the desired volume of cardioplegic solutions must be evenly distributed throughout the myocardium. Obstacles to this goal include coronary stenoses, which prevent uniform delivery of cardioplegia, often to the most vulnerable regions of the myocardium, and aortic regurgitation. Aortic regurgitation, even when mild, lowers aortic root pressure, so reducing the perfusion pressure of cardioplegia infused into the aortic root, and also causes loss of cardioplegia into the left ventricle. Hence, the time honored method of antegrade aortic root infusion of cardioplegia alone can be combined with "retrograde cardioplegia" infusion into the coronary sinus to overcome the potential for inadequate myocardial preservation.

Retrograde coronary venous cardioplegia perfusion via the coronary sinus overcomes the limitations of antegrade administration via the coronary arteries alone to ensure adequate left ventricular distribution of cardioplegia distal to coronary stenoses. Retrograde cardioplegia infusion is usually delivered via a balloon-tipped catheter inserted through the right atrium and guided into the coronary sinus. The balloon is either inflated manually or is self-inflating to prevent regurgitation of cardioplegia into the atrium. Retrograde infusion delivers cardioplegia uniformly throughout the left ventricle, but right ventricular coronary flow drains into veins more proximal to the catheter tip in the coronary sinus and thus retrograde cardioplegia does not protect the right ventricle. Many surgeons, therefore, use a combined method of antegrade and retrograde cardioplegia in most cardiac operations. In cases in which aortic regurgitation is manifest, cardioplegia may be infused directly into the coronary ostia by hand-held devices. A similar approach is used in other types of operations requiring opening of the aortic root for surgical access, e.g., for operations on the aorta.

## Antegrade delivery

Typically, a cannula for antegrade cardioplegia is placed high and slightly to the right side of the ascending aorta, secured with a purse-string suture, which is tied at the end of the operation. The cannula may include a pressure line and a vent port to suction air and blood between infusions. Antegrade infusion pressure during delivery of cardioplegia must be monitored. High pressures (>80 mmHg) may cause endothelial damage and myocardial edema. Monitoring pressure in the cardioplegia delivery system allows detection of inadvertent line occlusion by clamping or kinking. However, using the delivery system line pressure alone to estimate aortic or coronary sinus pressure is inaccurate. Accurate infusion pressure is obtained through a line directly attached to the infusion port. Such systems are widely available commercially.

Antegrade infusion pressure should be kept between 60 and 80 mmHg. High pressure during infusion is most likely to be due to extensive coronary stenotic lesions; the rate of infusion should be slowed to permit infusion of the required volume (usually 300 ml/minute for 2 minutes). If there is mild aortic insufficiency, antegrade cardioplegia will be infused partially into the left ventricle and will not be distributed into the myocardium very effectively. Light manual pressure applied to the right ventricle will often help close the left ventricular outflow tract. The perfusionist can confirm that cardioplegia is flowing into the myocardium by checking aortic root pressure and observing myocardial temperature change. Alternatively, the aortic root can be partially opened and cardioplegia directly infused into the coronary ostia using hand-held or self-inflating balloon catheters.

Further antegrade infusions of cardioplegia may be administered during CABG via the proximal ends of vein grafts on completion of each distal anastamosis.

## Retrograde delivery

A cannula for retrograde administration of cardioplegia is inserted through the lower part of the right atrium into the coronary sinus, usually before cardiopulmonary bypass is started. A cannula, designed for placement in the coronary sinus, with a malleable stylet and a self-inflating, or manually inflated, balloon is commonly used. The retrograde cannula is directed at a 45-degree angle towards the left shoulder in the path of the coronary sinus and positioned distally beneath the left atrial appendage. The cannula tip is palpated as it passes by the junction of the inferior vena cava and right atrium into the coronary sinus. If the cannula is directed into the posterior descending vein, it should be withdrawn slightly and reinserted. If difficulty is encountered during placement, it is helpful to commence CPB and lift the apex of the heart. The surgeon can then directly view and palpate the tip of the cannula making it easier to insert. In re-operations, if the posterior ventricular wall is adherent to the pericardium, placement of the retrograde cannula may be attempted prior to CPB, but may prove difficult. Alternatively, after CPB is instituted, adhesions can be dissected away from the heart and the cannula positioned more readily. Failure to intubate the coronary sinus is rare (under 2% of cases) and indicates a fenestrated thebesian valve or a flap over the coronary sinus ostium. When this occurs, bicaval cannulation may be used, permitting opening of the right atrium and direct insertion of the retrograde cannula into the ostium of the coronary sinus. During infusion of retrograde cardioplegia, the perfusionist should monitor the infusion pressure and reduce flow, if needed, so as not to exceed a pressure of about 40 mmHg. High pressures usually indicate that the catheter is advanced too far and should be withdrawn slightly.

The coronary sinus can be injured by forceful cannulation or continued infusion of cardioplegia with coronary sinus pressures exceeding 40 mmHg. Perforation of the sinus is manifest if an initially high coronary sinus pressure is followed by sudden low pressure, or by the surgeon noting blood within the pericardial well during cardioplegia infusions. Perforation can be directly repaired with a 5–0 suture or with pericardial pledgets if the tear site is not distinct. If a hematoma is noted, retrograde infusions should be discontinued. No further action is needed because low venous pressure allows self-containment after heparin reversal.

Coronary sinus pressure <20 mmHg infers that the balloon is not inflated or not occluding the coronary sinus. The catheter may have migrated out of the coronary sinus into the right atrium. The cannula tip and balloon should then be palpated and repositioned. Added maneuvers to improve retrograde infusion include finger compression of the junction of the coronary sinus and right atrium or placement of a snared suture around the coronary sinus, thus fixing it in place and preventing regurgitation of cardioplegia into the atrium. A rare cause of low retrograde infusion pressure is the presence of a left superior vena cava. This is usually determined before cardiopulmonary bypass and the vessel occluded with a tourniquet only if an intact innominate vein is present. If the innominate vein is absent, only antegrade cardioplegia is used.

## Cardioplegia temperature

Crystalloid cardioplegia solutions are usually delivered at 4°C, cold blood solutions at 10–16°C and warm blood solutions at 37°C.

Adequacy of cardioplegia distribution can be confirmed by monitoring myocardial temperature. The temperature probe can be placed in the septum first, the most vulnerable area, and then moved according to the surgeon's preferences to other regions of the heart. Temperature is generally kept below 15°C. Sometimes more cardioplegia needs to be infused to reach low temperatures, e.g., in the face of severe left ventricular hypertrophy commonly seen in hypertensive patients or in the setting of severe aortic stenosis. Inadequate cooling is sometimes seen if the two-staged venous cannula indirectly distorts the non-coronary cusp of the aortic valve, resulting in aortic regurgitation during cardioplegia infusion. Simply repositioning the cannula in the field will correct this problem.

Excessive blood accumulating in the heart during cardioplegic arrest leads to inadvertent myocardial re-warming and can be prevented by judicious use of vent suckers to drain the ventricles.

## Alternatives to cardioplegia

There are certain circumstances in which cardioplegia is not used in cardiac surgery. Fibrillatory arrest has been used for years and, though it is not advocated as a first-line method of myocardial protection, it is useful in special situations. One of the limitations of fibrillatory arrest is compression of the coronary vessels by the intensity of contraction of the fibrillating myocardium, which significantly impairs coronary blood flow. Systemic hypothermia to about 24°C reduces myocardial activity, and in association with maintaining systemic aortic pressure above 70 mmHg, may improve transmural perfusion pressure. Fibrillation, in conjunction with hypothermia and maintenance of a physiological level of perfusion pressure, can provide myocardial protection for periods of about an hour or more with reasonable recovery of global function. Utilization of this method of cold ventricular fibrillation is particularly useful during mitral valve repair or replacement in patients who have undergone prior coronary bypass grafting, in whom the risk of injury to patent grafts is to be avoided. CPB is instituted via femoral arterial and venous cannulation. The core temperature is reduced and the heart fibrillates at temperatures below 28°C. The left atrium can be entered via a limited right thoracotomy, providing the surgeon with an excellent view of the mitral valve. Aortic valve competence is necessary to prevent flooding of the operative field with blood. This method has been extensively reported and is commonly used during re-operative surgery.

## Optimum cardioplegic technique

Surgeons have advocated the merits of various manifestations of cardioplegia. There is ongoing controversy regarding the ideal composition, temperature (cold vs. warm), frequency of dosing and the route of administration (antegrade vs. retrograde) of cardioplegia.

The "integrated method" of cardioplegia administration is a technique that combines the advantages of many strategies while addressing the immediate needs of the myocardium during a cardiac operation. It hastens the recovery of the myocardium while not interfering with visualization during the cardiac operation. Coronary artery bypass is the most common cardiac operation, and so is used here to illustrate this example of the integrated method. Cardiopulmonary bypass is first initiated with cannulation of the aorta and right atrium and the core temperature is moderately reduced to about 34°C. The aorta is cross-clamped and the heart arrested with a cold cardioplegic mixture containing high-dose potassium (20 mEq/l) infused antegrade into the aortic root at a flow rate of 300 ml/minute for 2 minutes, followed by retrograde coronary sinus infusion at a flow rate of 200 ml/minute for 2 minutes. A diagram of a system used to deliver cold and warm cardioplegia via antegrade and retrograde routes and at low or high potassium strengths is shown in Figure 7.3.

Septal temperature is monitored with a temperature probe and usually falls to below 15°C. Topical hypothermia of the right ventricle may be supplemented with cold saline or iced saline slush with protection of the phrenic nerves to prevent postoperative palsy. This is not, however, mandatory. The right coronary is first grafted with saphenous vein. "Maintenance" low-dose cold potassium (8–10 mEq/l) blood cardioplegia is then infused simultaneously into the vein graft and coronary sinus at a flow rate of 200 ml/minute for 1 minute. The vein graft is then sewn onto the aorta while a continuous non-cardioplegic solution of modified cold blood is infused at 200 ml/minute. This "modified cold blood solution" (10°C) contains CPD, THAM, magnesium and mannitol and has been shown to provide better recovery than cold blood alone. The aorta is actively vented with suction applied to the cardioplegia catheter. The vent is discontinued and maintenance cardioplegia (low-dose cold potassium (8–10 mEq/l) blood cardioplegia) is infused into the aortic root at a flow of 200 ml/minute for 1 minute. After residual air is displaced from the aorta and as the cardioplegia blood emerges, the surgeon completes the anastamosis of the proximal end of the vein graft. The above procedure is repeated until all vein graft anastomoses, except one, are complete. After the last distal anastomosis is completed, the "hot shot" of warm substrate-enhanced cardioplegia is delivered, first antegrade into the ascending aorta at 150 ml/minute for 2 minutes, then retrograde through the coronary sinus and simultaneously through the last unattached saphenous

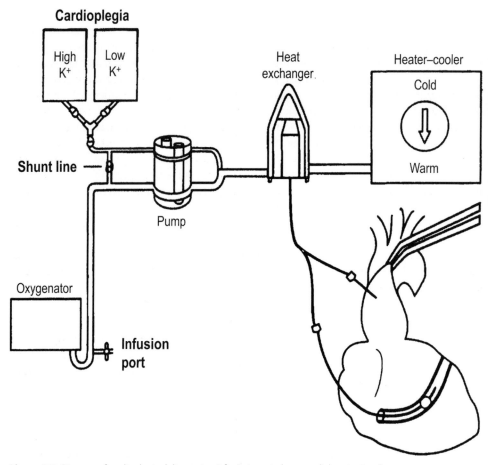

**Figure 7.3** Diagram of cardioplegia delivery circuit for "integrated myocardial protection."

vein graft proximal end at 150 ml/minute for 2 minutes. There is sometimes transient mild vasodilation due to the added amino acids and this is easily treated with neosynephrine (0.5 –1 µg/kg/minute). The final distal anastomosis is that of the internal mammary to the left anterior coronary artery. At this point the body and cardioplegia are re-warmed. As the last vein graft is sewn to the aorta, the cardioplegia is washed out of the myocardium by retrograde infusion of plain warm blood at a flow of 300 ml/minute. The heart begins contracting, slowly at first, then more rapidly and vigorously. The cardioplegia delivery system is turned to the antegrade mode of delivery and warm blood is infused into the aortic root while the aorta is still clamped for another 3–5 minutes. During this time, the perfusionist adjusts the flow to maintain an aortic root pressure of about 80 mmHg. Air is purged from the coronary grafts with a fine needle. The aortic clamp is then removed and the patient weaned off bypass, usually within 5 minutes with minimal (dopamine 2.5 µg/kg/minute) or no inotropic support in spite of lengthy aortic clamp times. Defibrillation is very rarely needed.

Note that the integrated method of protection involves a single period of aortic cross-clamping, which serves to limit atheroembolic events. Ischemic times are actually shortened in spite of longer clamp times and morbidity and cost have been shown to be reduced with this technique.

## Septal function

Impairment of the coordinated contraction of the interventricular septum is often apparent after cardiac operations. The "surgical septum" is a term echocardiographers use in describing the paradoxical movement of the septum seen in this context. A recent study of over 3000 cardiac surgical cases reported an incidence of approximately 40%. Interestingly, the septal dysfunction recovers with time in the majority of cases, but not all. Some believe the phenomenon of the "surgical septum" is normal after the pericardium is opened and is related to dissipation of the cardiac impulse in the absence of the tension provided by the closed pericardium. Alternatively, septal dysfunction may be viewed as a form of injury, either permanent or transient (stunning). Review of over 100 consecutive cardiac surgical procedures, including coronary bypass grafting and valve procedures with 2D echocardiography, has shown that septal dysfunction was absent in patients receiving "integrated myocardial protection." Protection of the septum may thus be a further advantage of the integrated technique. Prevention of septal dysfunction is crucial since the septum constitutes approximately one-third of the weight, and therefore structure, of the heart. Patients with reduced systolic function are particularly hemodynamically compromised immediately at the termination of CPB if septal contractility is also impaired.

## Cardioplegia in particular conditions

Under certain circumstances the technique of cardioplegia used ideally requires slight modifications based on the same general principles of protection. These circumstances include acute myocardial infarction and thoracic aortic aneurysms and examples of modifications that may be of benefit are described below.

## Evolving myocardial infarction

In patients with acute ischemia, or evolving myocardial infarction, the ventricle is ischemic and energy depleted because of lack of perfusion. The goal is to restore the depleted substrates and reverse ischemia by restoring flow with coronary grafts, while also preventing reperfusion injury to the myocardium. A substrate-enhanced low-potassium cardioplegia is used during these procedures, "acute MI/arrest" cardioplegia. This is a formulation that contains potassium to keep the heart arrested, a calcium channel blocker to prevent intracellular calcium influx and amino acid substrates to promote regeneration of high-energy phosphates. This solution is infused over a prolonged time (20 minutes). The normothermic arrested heart is replenished with the amino acid substrates aspartate and glutamate, which are rapidly assimilated into the myocardium to generate ATP needed for contractility.

Leukocyte depletion by adding filters to the cardioplegia in cases of acute infarction has also been shown to attenuate reperfusion injury.

## Myocardial protection during aortic root replacement

The myocardium must be carefully protected during aortic root replacement for dissection or aneurysmal disease. The coronary ostia are often surgically dissected and isolated for re-implantation into a prosthetic graft. Intermittent cardioplegia can be administered directly into these unattached ostia by hand-held cannulae or self-inflating balloon catheters, but care must be taken to avoid injury, particularly if operation is indicated because of dissection. An approach that has been found useful in cases of aortic dissection is first grafting the right coronary artery with saphenous vein. The proximal right coronary artery is temporarily occluded with a silastic vascular loop or soft jaw clamp. Cardioplegia can then be administered intermittently antegrade via the grafted right coronary artery for right ventricular protection and simultaneously retrograde into the coronary sinus for left ventricular protection. This permits excellent cardioplegia distribution throughout the myocardium and does not interfere with visualization during the operative procedure. The aortic root and ascending aorta can be replaced with ease in a dry field. After the root replacement, the saphenous vein graft is ligated at the anastomosis to the right coronary artery, either with a running suture or with a large hemoclip. The extra 5 minutes to execute this protective method ensures global myocardial protection and avoids injury to the friable coronary ostia.

## Conclusion

Blood cardioplegia is an effective and widely accepted method of myocardial protection. Retrograde cardioplegic delivery has been found to be useful in enhancing even distribution of cardioplegia, particularly distal to coronary stenoses in vessels supplying the left ventricular myocardium. Replenishment of substrates to the energy-depleted heart is a main focus of development for cardioplegia formulations, designed to enhance recovery following the ischemia required to carry out cardiac operations.

"Integrated myocardial management" is an easy and effective method of myocardial protection in adult cardiac procedures by expediting the operation and meeting the physiological needs of the myocardium. The duration of cardiopulmonary bypass is shortened by this technique by eliminating the need for recovery time following unclamping of the aorta. Excellent clinical outcomes have been reported and this method has been employed in many centers for several years.

Ongoing studies are needed to develop additional cardioprotective strategies. These may include the use of preconditioning agents, white blood cell filters, free radical scavengers and endothelium-enhancing agents.

## Suggested Further Reading

- Allen BS, Okamoto F, Buckberg GD, et al. Immediate functional recovery after six hours of regional ischemia by careful control of conditions of reperfusion and composition of reperfusate. *J Thorac Cardiovasc Surg* 1986; **92**: 621–35.

- Athanasuleas C, Siler W, Buckberg G. Myocardial protection during surgical ventricular restoration. *Eur J Cardiothorac Surg* 2006; **29** (Suppl 1): S231–7.

- Beyersdorf F, Acar C, Buckberg GD, et al. Studies on prolonged acute regional ischemia. III. Early natural history of simulated single and multivessel disease with emphasis on remote myocardium. *J Thorac Cardiovasc Surg* 1989; **98**: 368–80.

- Buckberg GD, Beyersdorf F, Allen BS, Robertson JM. Integrated myocardial management: background and initial application. *J Card Surg* 1995; **10**: 68–89.

- Buckberg GD. Development of blood cardioplegia and retrograde techniques: the experimenter/observer complex. *J Card Surg* 1998; **13**: 163–70.

- Ihnken K, Morita K, Buckberg GD, et al. Simultaneous arterial and coronary sinus cardioplegic perfusion: an experimental and clinical study. *J Thorac Cardiovasc Surg* 1994; **42**: 141–7.

- Loop FD, Higgins TL, Panda R, Pearce G, Estafanous FG. Myocardial protection during cardiac operations: decreased morbidity and lower cost with blood cardioplegia and coronary sinus perfusion. *J Thorac Cardiovasc Surg* 1992; **104**: 608–18.

- Noyez L, van Son JA, van der Werf T, et al. Retrograde versus antegrade delivery of cardioplegic solution in myocardial revascularization: a clinical trial in patients with three-vessel coronary artery disease who underwent myocardial revascularization with extensive use of the internal mammary artery. *J Thorac Cardiovasc Surg* 1993; **105**: 854–63.

- Partington MT, Acar C, Buckberg GD, Julia PL. Studies of retrograde cardioplegia. II. Advantages of antegrade/retrograde cardioplegia to optimize distribution in jeopardized myocardium. *J Thorac Cardiovasc Surg* 1989; **97**: 613–22.

- Teoh KH, Christakis GT, Weisel RD, *et al.* Accelerated myocardial metabolic recovery with terminal warm blood cardioplegia. *J Thorac Cardiovasc Surg* 1986; **91**: 888–95.

**Chapter 8**

# Weaning from cardiopulmonary bypass

James Keogh, Susanna Price and Brian Keogh

Weaning, the process of transition from cardiopulmonary bypass (CPB) to normal, physiological circulation, requires excellent communication and teamwork between perfusionist, surgeon and anesthetist. Numerous mechanical, physiological and pharmacological factors need to be efficiently coordinated within an extremely short time frame. Weaning passes smoothly in the majority of cases and, as such, is often viewed as a routine process. In patients with pre-existing poor or borderline cardiac function, or in whom unexpected difficulties are encountered, weaning from CPB may prove complex, but should not impede the patient's progression to recovery. By contrast, if the weaning process is poorly managed, or if warning signs of deterioration are missed, complications encountered during the weaning phase may, of themselves, contribute additional morbidity.

## Preparation

Separation from CPB requires the heart to resume its function as the driving force of blood flow, taking over from the mechanical pump in the CPB circuit. In order to achieve a smooth transition, cardiac function must be optimized prior to weaning from CPB. Delays in investigating or treating abnormal parameters may lead to the heart failing, necessitating a return to extracorporeal circulation. Consequently, anticipation of possible cardiac dysfunction and thorough advance preparation are key elements of the weaning process. A checklist of physiological parameters that should be optimized prior to weaning is given in Table 8.1 and discussed below.

## Temperature

Re-warming to a core temperature above 36°C is the first step in weaning from CPB. In addition to multiple temperature monitoring sites on the bypass machine, which should include blood temperature and the temperature of the heat exchanger, body temperature may be monitored at a number of sites, for example nasopharyngeal, esophageal, intracardiac, bladder or rectum. It is important to appreciate that re-warming is not uniform and the determination of which site (or sites) best represents adequate re-warming will vary according to how much the patient has been cooled, the duration of hypothermic bypass and patient considerations, such as body surface area. A combination of bladder temperature and the temperature of the venous blood returning to the bypass circuit is particularly valuable when CPB temperature has been below 30°C. Active surface warming using a forced warm air device should be combined with re-warming via the extracorporeal circuit to reduce redistribution of heat from core to peripheral tissues. If re-warming is inadequate, or if the core-surface gradient is greater than 7°C, significant further heat loss may occur during wound closure. Shivering and increased peripheral vascular resistance in the recovery period will result in

**Table 8.1.** Preparation for weaning from cardiopulmonary bypass

| |
|---|
| Re-warm to target temperatures |
| Correct electrolytes and acid–base |
| Achieve target hemoglobin |
| Ensure access to blood and blood products |
| Establish vasoactive support infusions |
| Prepare anesthesia transition |
| Assess rate, rhythm and conduction |
| Control arrhythmias |
| Establish pacing as required |
| TOE functioning if employed |
| Additional techniques if difficulty predicted |

an unwanted increase in oxygen consumption. Conversely, core temperature should not be allowed to rise above 37°C as this will lead to tachycardia and may increase the risk of central nervous system dysfunction.

# Electrolytes and acid/base

Electrolyte abnormalities should be corrected before separation from CPB in order to optimize myocyte function. In particular, potassium, magnesium and calcium should be kept within the normal range.

- **Potassium** (4.0–5.5 mmol/l) – Hypokalemia can cause arrhythmia and should be treated if below 4 mmol/l. In many centers potassium is maintained at the "higher" end of the normal range in order to suppress the development of arrhythmias, to which the heart is particularly susceptible in the early post-CPB phase. Hyperkalemia can cause conduction abnormalities and impair contractility. Values above 6.0 mmol/l should serve as an alert to monitor biochemical parameters closely and levels above 6.5 mmol/l should be actively treated before weaning.
- **Calcium** (1.09–1.30 mmol/l) – The concentration of calcium in the plasma may be reduced by large volumes of citrated blood, leading to impaired contractility and vasodilatation. Ionized calcium should be maintained above 1.0 mmol/l.
- **Magnesium** (0.80–1.40 mmol/l) – Low levels of magnesium are associated with dysrhythmia and should be corrected below 0.7 mmol/l. It is worth noting that some point-of-care analyzers, notably the Nova Biomedical range, employ a lower range measuring ionized magnesium, so it is important to check the nature of the measurement and the device normal range before interpreting the result.
- **Glucose** (4.0–7.8 mmol/l) – Tight glucose control in the postoperative period has been shown by some investigators to improve outcome after cardiac surgery and investigation of its impact in the perioperative phase is ongoing. Extrapolation of the available evidence and majority practice suggest that significant hyperglycemia (>12 mmol/l) should be treated with an insulin infusion, although treatment thresholds remain varied. Hypoglycemia in association with CPB is extremely rare in the absence of liver failure and, if encountered, should be judiciously treated and its cause investigated.

- **Lactate** (0.7–2.5 mmol/l) – Elevated serum lactate levels are commonly encountered during prolonged episodes of CPB, particularly if there have been periods of low pump flow or if circulatory arrest has been employed. Treatment of lactic acidosis per se is not usually instituted but the value should be noted and any progression seen as a potential indicator of inadequate organ perfusion.
- **Metabolic acidosis** – This is also commonly observed during CPB and there are differing approaches to its correction. Some units very tightly correct base deficits to baseline whereas the majority of units readily accept base deficits of up to –5 mmol/l. Most teams would treat a base deficit in excess of –10 mmol/l. Between these values, debate about treatment thresholds in this context continues.

## Hemoglobin

For most patients, the hemoglobin concentration should be above 7.5 g/dl prior to termination of CPB. In situations where myocardial oxygen supply or whole body oxygen delivery are expected to be impaired post-CPB, for example residual coronary stenosis or low cardiac output states, it is preferable to aim for a higher hemoglobin concentration. Similarly, when bleeding is expected to be an ongoing problem in the post-CPB period, hemoglobin should be maintained at a higher level. Comorbid pathology, particularly coexisting respiratory disease, may also indicate the need for a higher hemoglobin level at weaning. In patients with congenital heart disease who remain cyanosed after surgery, a higher hemoglobin concentration is mandatory.

Stored, concentrated red blood cells should be immediately accessible for use in the post-bypass period. In the majority of cases, cell salvaged blood should ideally become available within 10–15 minutes of weaning from CPB, thus reducing the need for use of stored "bank" blood in the first instance.

## Coagulation

Due to the nature of cardiac surgery, particularly the anticoagulation required and the effects of the extracorporeal circuit on the clotting cascade and platelet function, patients undergoing CPB are at significant risk of bleeding. Consequently, ready access to serum clotting factors and platelets must be ensured. Following separation from CPB and reversal of anticoagulation, assessment of clotting and platelet function should be performed according to unit protocols (laboratory-based clotting screen, activated clotting time, heparin assays or thromboelastography (TEG)). Persistent surgical bleeding and the absence of visible clot formation should initiate blood product support, informed by coagulation measurements. It is, however, important to emphasize that abnormal clotting assessments alone should not initiate blood product administration in the operating theater if the surgical field does not show evidence of ongoing bleeding.

## Volume

In addition to ready access to blood products, colloid and crystalloid solutions should be immediately available to increase circulating volume when indicated.

## Vasoactive drugs

Vasopressors, inotropes and vasodilators must be immediately to hand, if not already prepared and loaded onto infusion pumps, primed for use. The choice of agents should be based on the patient's circulation, nature of the surgery and local team protocols. The vasoactive support strategy should be agreed by the team before weaning from CPB commences.

## Anesthesia

Anesthesia, analgesia and neuromuscular blockade must be assessed and supplemented as required. Weaning from CPB may instigate either a change in anesthetic technique (e.g., intravenous to volatile) or an adjustment to dose delivery. Regardless of the exact nature of this change, it is vital that anesthesia is properly maintained and this should be confirmed by the team members.

## Cardiac function

Following unclamping of the aorta an adequate reperfusion period must be permitted. This allows the heart to replenish metabolic substrates, specifically high-energy phosphates (ATP), and "washes out" the products of anaerobic metabolism, before attempting to wean from CPB. A commonly employed rule is 20 minutes of reperfusion for every hour of ischemic (aortic cross-clamp) time, although practice is varied. Surgical sequence may facilitate this myocardial resuscitative period – for example, right-sided surgery (e.g., tricuspid annuloplasty) or the aortic anastomoses of coronary revascularization grafts may be performed during the reperfusion period.

Cardiac function should be assessed as far as possible prior to weaning from CPB. This assessment should concentrate on three main areas: rate, rhythm and contractility. Following CPB, the ventricles are generally less compliant and will not have the normal capacity to increase stroke volume. Heart rate is therefore usually maintained at between 80 and 100 beats per minute to partially compensate for this. Another result of a stiff ventricle is an increase in the relative importance of the contribution of atrial contraction to stroke volume and consequently sinus rhythm is always preferable if possible. Epicardial pacing leads and an external pacemaker should always be immediately available, ideally with dual chamber function to allow sequential atrio-ventricular pacing.

Contractility can be assessed by direct visualization of the right ventricle. If in use, transesophageal echocardiography (TOE) enables a more detailed examination of all four chambers. If any of the cardiac chambers have been opened during the procedure, for example in valve replacement surgery, it is essential to evacuate any air from the heart prior to separation from bypass.

## Predicting difficulty

Occasionally, despite careful preparation, weaning from CPB is difficult, and the identification of patients who will present a particular challenge allows additional preparations to be made in advance.

Commonly encountered risk factors for failure to wean from CPB include:

- poor preoperative ventricular function;
- urgent and emergency surgery;
- prolonged aortic cross-clamp time;
- inadequate myocardial protection; and
- incomplete surgical repair.

When faced with a high-risk patient there are several strategies that can be employed. An intra-aortic balloon pump may be inserted before the start of surgery in patients with poor ventricular function. Inotropes and vasopressors can be commenced at re-warming, ensuring they have cleared the dead-space of administration lines prior to weaning from CPB. If inotropes require administration of a loading dose (e.g., milrinone, levosimendan), these should ideally be given after aortic unclamping, during re-warming. Dilute solutions of adrenaline (epinephrine) or noradrenaline (norepinephrine) can be prepared to allow delivery of small boluses to aid evaluation of the response of the myocardium.

If sinus rhythm is not re-established, or supraventricular arrythmias or ventricular irritability is observed despite correction of metabolic parameters, anti-arrhythmic therapy should be prepared and administered as necessary, well before weaning from CPB is attempted. Electrical cardioversion may be required in isolation, or in addition to anti-arrhythmic agents.

Additional invasive monitoring lines may be prepared, permitting direct measurement of cardiac chamber pressures and valve gradients. These lines may additionally be used later for administration of protamine into the left side of the heart, thus attenuating the pulmonary hypertensive response (see below).

## Events immediately prior to initiating weaning

### Mechanical ventilation

During CPB the lungs are allowed to deflate fully or to remain slightly inflated at low levels of positive end expiratory pressure (PEEP). As a result there will be widespread alveolar collapse. Prior to weaning from CPB full and effective expansion of the lungs should be ensured, usually with manual hyperinflation. If one or both pleural cavities are open, visualization of the lung is facilitated and the pleural cavities may be drained of any accumulated fluid. Once expansion is achieved, mechanical ventilation is resumed, usually with PEEP. It is prudent to apply tracheo-bronchial suction to the lungs to clear any excess respiratory secretions.

Effective mechanical ventilation of the lungs must be ensured prior to commencing weaning from CPB. Ventilation should be initiated when it no longer interferes with surgical maneuvers, and in any case when there are signs of significant left ventricular ejection; cardiac ejection while on CPB in the presence of a competent aortic valve suggests re-establishment of significant pulmonary blood flow. If the lungs remain unventilated, this pulmonary blood flow will acts as a true right to left shunt, delivering deoxygenated blood to the left ventricle. This deoxygenated blood will then be ejected and mixed with oxygenated blood from the aortic cannula and, depending on the volume of ejected blood, may result in undesirable systemic arterial hypoxia in the latter stages of CPB.

The perfusionist and anesthetist must confirm to each other that effective ventilation has been resumed. The consequence of weaning from CPB without ventilation is the rapid onset of hypoxia, followed by bradycardia, cardiac failure and organ damage.

### Physiological alarms

Alarms settings for many parameters displayed on anesthetic monitors and ventilators are greatly modified or even disabled during CPB. It is vital that physiological monitoring with appropriate alarm settings is re-enabled prior to weaning from CPB. This should be seen as a team responsibility rather than that of an individual, and the anesthetist and perfusionist should specifically confirm that physiological and ventilation monitoring have been re-enabled prior to commencing weaning.

## Arterial blood gases and electrolytes

Following re-warming, an arterial blood gas and electrolytes sample should be taken, reviewed by the team and appropriate measures taken. In the majority of cases little or no corrective action is required. The commonest adjustments that need to be made are to acid–base status and potassium levels.

Metabolic acidosis may require treatment according to local protocols. Sodium bicarbonate ($NaHCO_3$) is commonly administered to correct the acidosis. Administration of sodium bicarbonate solution, usually into the cardiotomy reservoir of the extracorporeal circuit, generates a substantial amount of intracellular carbon dioxide and is often associated with a reduction in systemic vascular resistance. Although cardiac myocytes are thought to have effective intracellular buffering mechanisms, the administration of a large volume of sodium bicarbonate in a short period may generate paradoxical intracellular acidosis. Clearance of this excess generated carbon dioxide via the oxygenator membrane may take 5–10 minutes and can be monitored by a return to baseline of oxygenator exhaust capnography levels or less obviously by in-line blood carbon dioxide tension. Most importantly, in patients with poor cardiac function, and in particular poor right ventricular function, weaning from CPB should not be attempted until the risk of significant paradoxical intracellular acidosis has passed and the majority of excess carbon dioxide has been cleared.

As previously discussed, serum values of potassium and ionized calcium should be normalized. Magnesium is increasingly popular as an anti-arrhythmic agent and may be administered following aortic de-clamping regardless of the baseline serum level. A bolus of $MgSO_4$ can cause profound vasodilatation; the systemic vascular resistance should be allowed to recover, or vasoconstrictors administered, prior to weaning from CPB. In general, magnesium is best administered soon after aortic unclamping.

## De-airing of the heart

Any cardiac surgical procedure that requires opening of cardiac chambers will inevitably allow introduction of air. Air in right-sided chambers is usually innocuous as long as its volume is not substantial enough to prevent forward flow and provided there are no breaches in the atrial or ventricular septum. Air in the left side is dangerous and presents two major risks:

- cerebral air embolus with postoperative morbidity, ranging from minimal transient confusion to widespread neurological damage; and
- coronary air embolus, which may cause transient and possibly widespread regional ventricular dysfunction and, in the extreme, irreversible myocardial damage.

It is therefore vital that meticulous attention to de-airing is applied. Direct cardiac massage and syringing of left-sided chambers and venting of the aorta or left-sided chambers is best undertaken in a head down position, prior to, and after, aortic unclamping. It is customary to ventilate the lungs during the de-airing process in order to displace air that accumulates in the pulmonary veins. Indeed, such air may arise from the pulmonary veins even if the left-sided chambers are not opened, although its degree is usually limited in this context. The introduction of TOE into cardiac practice has greatly improved the de-airing process, allowing targeting of air "pockets" and de-airing until the amount of residual intracardiac air is considered acceptable (Figure 8.1).

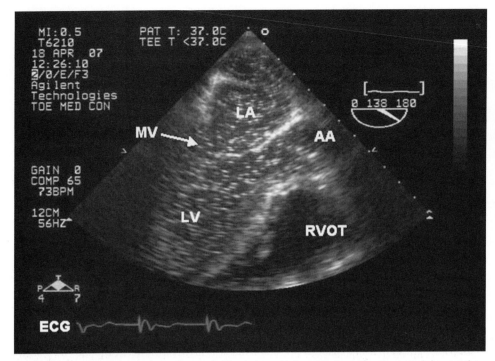

**Figure 8.1** Trans-esophageal echocardiogram (mid-esophageal, left ventricular outflow tract view) showing the heart during de-airing following aortic valve surgery. Air is seen as white speckles throughout the left heart. Of note, there is no air seen in the right heart. AA = ascending aorta; ECG = electrocardiogram; LA = left atrium; LV = left ventricle; MV = mitral valve (arrowed); RVOT = right ventricular outflow tract.

## Epicardial pacing

Epicardial pacing is commonly required in the immediate and early post-CPB period. Atrial pacing may be used alone to increase heart rate in patients in sinus rhythm or in a junctional rhythm in which atrio-ventricular (A-V) conduction is intact. When possible, atrial pacing is preferable to A-V or ventricular pacing. Ventricular pacing may be employed in isolation when there is no effective atrial contraction (e.g., in chronic atrial fibrillation). In cases in which A-V synchronization is likely to be helpful and effective sinus rhythm is not established, atrial and ventricular epicardial leads should be placed to facilitate sequential A-V pacing. Sequential pacing, usually using atrial and right ventricular leads, may also be established in atrio-left ventricular or atrio-biventricular (with right and left ventricular leads) fashion. The latter is analogous to the application of cardiac re-synchronization therapy. This intervention may result in a rapid increase in cardiac output of up to 30% and is increasingly employed in patients with poor left ventricular function following, or as an aide to, weaning from CPB.

Epicardial pacing is usually established prior to weaning from CPB so that its benefits can be harnessed during that process. Some surgeons, however, prefer to wean from CPB with ventricular pacing alone and to secure atrial pacing leads after the venous cannulae have been removed. The pacing system and pacing and sensing thresholds should be tested prior to weaning.

Establishment of an appropriate mode of epicardial pacing is specifically intended to improve cardiac performance. Commonly, pacing is usually set at around 80–90 bpm immediately post-CPB. However, the pacing rate should be determined by patient needs and not strictly by protocol. When using dual chamber pacing, the standard preset atrio-ventricular interval is usually 150 ms; however, where increased heart rates are required, the A-V delay should be adjusted accordingly.

If cardiac function is adequate after weaning from CPB, pacing may not prove necessary.

## Mechanics of separation from CPB

On confirmation that cardiovascular, respiratory and metabolic parameters are within satis-factory limits and that the patient is adequately re-warmed and ventilated, the perfusionist commences weaning, initially by incrementally occluding venous return to the CPB circuit, thus allowing cardiac filling. The arterial pump flow is gradually reduced. If cardiac ejection progressively increases to a level considered suitable for maintenance of physiological circula-tion, the venous return pipe is completely occluded, the arterial flow reduced to "off" and the transition from CPB to "normal" circulation completed.

At this stage, in an ideal situation, the heart should be relatively relaxed and empty, both left and right atrial filling pressures low (2–5 mmHg). Ventricular filling can be further enhanced, if required, by infusion of fluid via the aortic cannula (in adults, usually in 100 ml aliquots). Conventional teaching is that the heart should be weaned from CPB with low filling pressures, allowing both ventricles time to accommodate to working under the increasing ventricular end-diastolic pressures associated with changes in pre- and afterload.

Weaning from CPB may take literally a few seconds in a patient with vigorous cardiac action who might typically be taken to "half-flow" and then "off" within moments. In patients with less promising cardiac function, the weaning process may be considerably protracted, necessitating a period of "partial bypass," that is, low-flow CPB, during which time titration of ventricular volume loading and optimization of inotropes, vasoconstrictors and cardiac rhythm can be undertaken.

### Assessment and adjustment of preload

Central venous pressure, in the context of the arterial pressures generated, guides the degree of filling of the heart. Perfusionists rarely have the opportunity to inspect the external appear-ance of the heart, which provides considerable information to surgeon and anesthetist. Nor-mally, the right ventricle only is observed: a comfortable, relaxed and slightly underfilled right ventricle typically displays inward dimpling of its anterior surface during systole. In patients with impaired left ventricular function, or if weaning from CPB is proving difficult, direct left atrial pressure or pulmonary artery/pulmonary capillary wedge pressure measurements are helpful. In some centers, all patients presenting for cardiac surgery have both central venous and pulmonary artery catheters placed perioperatively.

Surgeons typically also use pulmonary artery palpation, which reflects left atrial pres-sure, to guide left ventricular filling. TOE, when available, helps to assess preload and may be particularly useful in the presence of restrictive ventricular physiology, when higher filling pressures may be encountered at lower ventricular cavity volumes.

### Assessment of contractility and inotropic support

Considerable information about myocardial contractility can be gleaned from observing the heart. Well-coordinated contraction generating an acceptable aortic pulsation to meet desired arterial blood pressure targets suggests an acceptable inotropic state. Additionally, a reasonably sharp upstroke in the monitored arterial wave (dp/dt) and wide area under the arterial waveform curve are also indicative of contractility, but are also dependent on pre- and afterload. Quantitative measures of contractility include thermodilution or alternative cardiac output evaluation techniques; these delineate values for stroke volume if the heart rate is known. The information that TOE can provide about ventricular function is usually qualitative, but technology is evolving to provide readily interpretable quantitative echocardiographic analyses of myocardial contractility.

Inotropic support should be adjusted using the best information available about the patient's cardiovascular status. The strategies employed are considered below and generally guided by institutional and local team practice. Inotropic support should, if possible, be optimized during the period of weaning from CPB, giving the patient with borderline cardiac function the best conditions for a successful transition from CPB.

## Assessment of afterload

Systemic vascular resistance (SVR) values are usually assumed to be low following CPB because of the association between hemodilution and reduction in SVR and because of the systemic inflammatory response accompanying CPB. Patients at risk of a profound inflammatory response include those with long CPB times, long aortic cross-clamp times, complex surgery and previous exposure to CPB. It is therefore common for short-acting vasoconstrictors (e.g., metaraminol, phenylephrine) to be administered during CPB and in the weaning phase. Similarly, infusions of noradrenaline (norepinephrine) or vasopressin (ADH) are commonly administered to maintain SVR in the post-CPB period.

A reasonable estimate of systemic vascular resistance can be obtained while on CPB using the equation:

$$[\text{MAP (mmHg)} - \text{RA (mmHg)}]/\text{pump flow (l/min)} = \text{SVR (Wood Units)}$$

This is accurate unless there is additional native cardiac output, in which case the equation will overestimate the SVR, since the denominator will be falsely low. Wood units of vascular resistance are converted to more commonly used international units (dyn.s/cm$^5$) by multiplying the Wood unit value by 80.

Normal values for SVR are 900–1200 dyn.s/cm$^5$. Units of SVR are sometimes indexed to body surface area.

As a wide range of conditions is encountered in cardiac surgical practice, optimal SVR for weaning from CPB needs to be individually considered according to pathophysiology. However, the following considerations generally apply:

- patients with dilated, poorly functioning left ventricles, exhibiting a low ejection fraction (<30%), are thought to benefit from lower range SVR values;
- patients with coronary disease with residual, flow-limiting lesions or with left ventricular hypertrophy with small cavity size, but normal cardiac outputs, are thought to benefit from SVR values higher than normal; and
- coexisting disease in other organs, particularly cerebral or renal, may also dictate the requirement for higher SVR in order to maintain adequate perfusion pressures to these organs.

Consideration must also be given to the anesthetic protocol employed. Anesthesia based on delivery of volatile agents, prior to and during extracorporeal circulation, typically results in low SVR values (700–900 dyn.s/cm$^5$) when the patient is fully re-warmed. Older, intravenous agent-based protocols (e.g., high-dose opioids plus benzodiazepines) usually result in

**Table 8.2.** Sequence of events prior to weaning from cardiopulmonary bypass

| |
|---|
| Confirm effective ventilation |
| Re-enable physiological alarms |
| Final check of electrolytes and acid–base status |
| Correct acidosis if required |
| Effective de-airing of heart |
| Confirm satisfactory pacing lead thresholds |
| Confirm vasoactive agent delivery |
| Engage all team members |

**Table 8.3.** Key benefits of TOE when weaning from cardiopulmonary bypass

| |
|---|
| Confirm adequate de-airing |
| Guide filling and manipulation of preload |
| Confirm valve integrity and function |
| Identify para-prosthetic leaks |
| Confirm outflow tracts unobstructed |
| Display ventricular and septal movement |
| Identify regional wall abnormalities |
| Identify global ventricular dysfunction |
| Identify restrictive ventricular filling |
| Optimize pacing settings |
| Guide manipulation of contractility |

values twice that level. The use of propofol infusions during CPB often result in lesser reduction in SVR than seen with volatile agents.

The steps to be taken immediately before attempting to wean a patient off CPB are summarized in Table 8.2.

# The role of TOE in weaning from CPB

Intraoperative TOE has an increasing role in cardiac surgical procedures. There is institutional variation in the use of this tool in adult cardiac surgery, varying from its routine through to highly selective application. If difficulties are encountered in weaning from CPB, and particularly if they are unexpected, TOE can be an extremely valuable tool in informed decision making.

A detailed examination of the role of TOE is beyond the scope of this chapter. A limited summary of key benefits specific to intraoperative weaning from CPB is given in Table 8.3.

# Reversal of anticoagulation

To reverse heparinization, protamine is administered after successful transition from CPB to physiological circulation. Practice of heparin reversal varies among centers:

- a fixed dose based on the patient's weight (usually 3–4 mg/kg) can be given regardless of the heparin dose; or

- the protamine dose is titrated to the amount of heparin given, usually 1.0–1.3 mg protamine for each 100 units of heparin administered.

The venous cannulae are removed prior to protamine administration and the arterial cannula is removed either prior to, during or after protamine is given, according to local practice. Preload can be supported during protamine administration by titrated fluid administration from the extracorporeal circuit whilst the arterial cannula is *in situ*.

Protamine administration may be associated with circulatory instability due to unwanted vasoactive effects. They are usually limited to mild or moderate vasodilatation and mild negative inotropic effects, which can normally be attenuated by slow administration of protamine over 5–15 minutes. More severe adverse reactions to protamine can be expected in patients with existing pulmonary hypertension, due to its pulmonary vasoconstrictive effects. In a small number of patients, and more likely following previous cardiac surgery, adverse hemodynamic responses may be unexpectedly severe, some representing anaphylactoid or, in extreme cases, anaphylactic responses to protamine or the protamine–heparin complex. These rare but severe responses require escalation of inotropic and vasoconstrictor support. Use of pulmonary vasodilators may be necessary and, in exceptional cases, return to CPB may be the course of safety whilst measures to augment cardiovascular performance are instituted.

# Failure to achieve satisfactory weaning from CPB

## Reinstitution of CPB

Attempted weaning from CPB immediately resulting in unsatisfactory hemodynamic parameters, or followed by a gradual decline in cardiovascular status, should prompt consideration of a return to CPB, particularly if the hemodynamic deterioration is catastrophic or unexpected.

Reinstitution of CPB should not necessarily be seen as an adverse event. Although it will inevitably result in a prolongation of the total CPB time, it will allow:

- escalation of monitoring (e.g., left atrial line, pulmonary artery catheter);
- time for optimization of drug therapy and confirmation of drug delivery;
- fine tuning of hematocrit, acid–base and electrolyte status;
- checking the integrity of surgical intervention (e.g., eliminate kinked coronary bypass grafts, paraprosthetic leaks); and
- identification of other reversible causes of myocardial failure.

It is occasionally necessary to return to CPB due to major bleeding, such as dehiscence of a surgical anastamosis, correction of which might not be possible off-CPB.

An intra-aortic balloon pump may be inserted during this period and the team should have a low threshold for employing this option if there is persistent myocardial failure not readily reversible by less invasive measures.

## Vasopressors and inotropes – choices in weaning from CPB

Hypotension caused by reduction in SVR post-CPB may result in impaired coronary blood flow and myocardial ischemia. In this situation, a vasopressor such as noradrenaline (norepinephrine), vasopressin or phenylephrine is indicated.

Low cardiac output syndrome after cardiopulmonary bypass is multifactorial, but potential causes include pre-existing ventricular dysfunction, residual myocardial ischemia, inadequate myocardial protection, prolonged cross-clamp time with reperfusion injury, arrhythmia, activation of inflammatory cascades and imperfect surgical repair. Reversible causes for cardiac failure should be identified, treated appropriately and inotropic support instituted as necessary.

Inotropic drugs improve ventricular performance at the cost of increasing myocardial oxygen demand. Their use in the early post-CPB period should ideally be guided by objective measurements of cardiac performance such as left atrial pressure (reflecting left ventricular end-diastolic pressure, in the absence of mitral valve disease), cardiac output monitoring, pulmonary capillary wedge pressure measurement or TOE.

There are considerable variations in pharmacological strategies employed by cardiothoracic teams in weaning from CPB. As yet there is no clear evidence for the use of any one inotropic drug or combination of drugs over any other.

The main options for acute inotropic support during weaning from CPB are:

- **Adrenaline** (epinephrine) – A naturally occurring catecholamine with both alpha and beta receptor activity leading to increased intracellular cyclic AMP and protein kinase C activity. Adrenaline increases cardiac output by increasing contractility and heart rate, and is frequently employed in moderately to severely impaired contractility. It may be administered during weaning as a bolus injection to rapidly stimulate increased ventricular contractility. At high continuous infusion doses it may cause considerable vasoconstriction and raised serum lactate.
- **Dopamine** – A naturally occurring catecholamine that binds to both alpha and beta adrenergic receptors. Beta effects tend to predominate at low doses with alpha effects more prominent at high doses. Dopamine increases cardiac output by increasing heart rate and contractility; however, at higher doses blood pressure may be increased by raising systemic vascular resistance with no increase in cardiac output. Dopamine is generally used in more mild impairment of hemodynamics. There is no evidence to confirm the role of dopamine as a "renal protective drug."
- **Dobutamine** – A synthetic catecholamine and derivative of isoprenaline, dobutamine possesses strong affinity to beta receptors with little alpha activity. Contractility and heart rate are increased along with a reduction in systemic vascular resistance, leading to a rise in cardiac output. At higher doses the effects on heart rate tend to predominate and may limit its use in moderate cardiac failure. Its use in weaning from CPB appears to have waned with the availability of phosphodiesterase inhibitors.
- **Milrinone, enoximone** – Often referred to as "inodilators," these are bipyridine phosphodiesterase-III (PDE III) inhibitors, which exert their effects by inhibiting the breakdown of intracellular cyclic AMP and thus increasing stores of the high-energy phosphate, ATP. PDE III inhibitors improve contractility, increase heart rate and cause systemic and pulmonary vasodilatation. PDE III inhibitors appear to be associated with a lower incidence of tachycardia and arrhythmia than beta-agonists and tolerance is not a feature, but they may need to be administered with a vasoconstrictor. There is some evidence that prophylactic use of PDE III inhibitors prior to separation from cardiopulmonary bypass improves the chances of successful weaning and reduces the incidence of low cardiac output syndrome postoperatively.
- **Levosimendan** – This is another class of inodilator, which binds to cardiac troponin C, enhancing the myofilament responsiveness to calcium. Early studies suggest levosimendan is more effective at improving cardiac performance than dobutamine, but experience and information available in the literature remain limited.

# Functional mitral regurgitation

Acute mitral regurgitation in a patient with a morphologically normal mitral valve is occasionally encountered during and after weaning from CPB. Although infrequent, it usually occurs in patients undergoing coronary revascularization. This phenomenon, functional mitral regurgitation, is readily treatable with an excellent outcome, but can be surprisingly difficult to identify. Failure to recognize and treat it appropriately may lead to considerable morbidity.

As mentioned previously, weaning from CPB should be accomplished with a low ventricular filling volume and pressure, allowing the heart time to accommodate to the changing loading conditions. If CPB is terminated rapidly with high venous pressures and ventricular volumes, the left ventricle may become relatively ischemic and dilate. As a result the mitral valve annulus will be stretched, rendering the mitral valve acutely incompetent; the right ventricle faces acute left atrial hypertension and will appear characteristically dilated and domed, with limited contraction and no effective dimpling of its anterior surface. More commonly than this sudden scenario, the development of functional mitral regurgitation is insidious and the result of overzealous fluid infusion to treat low systemic arterial pressures. A further fluid challenge in this state characteristically results in a fall in systemic pressure. Adrenaline administration may increase the systemic diastolic pressure through vasoconstriction, but usually makes both the mitral regurgitant fraction and oxygen demand of the left ventricle much worse. Typically, even in a patient with previously preserved left ventricular function, systemic hypotension intractably persists and the condition rapidly becomes a medical emergency. The diagnosis is confirmed by TOE, if available, but the condition occurs typically in patients with low-grade indication for TOE. In the absence of TOE in situ, it is confirmed by direct left atrial pressure measurement, characteristically displaying a peak mitral regurgitant systolic wave of the order of 50–70 mmHg.

The treatment for functional mitral regurgitation is venodilatation, using nitroglycerine (GTN) or sodium nitroprusside, to rapidly reduce the left ventricular end-diastolic volume. Venodilatation is inevitably accompanied by arteriolar vasodilatation and, as effective coronary blood flow must be restored, aggressive venodilatation should be followed by a short-acting vasoconstrictor. The administration of a venodilator to a patient with a mean arterial pressure of 40–50 mmHg may appear counterintuitive, and brave, but is supported by an understanding of the pathophysiology. It is necessary to first reduce ventricular volume and shrink the mitral valve annulus and then support coronary perfusion to the ventricle by raising systemic pressure.

Alternative surgical approaches to the management of functional mitral regurgitation may include rapidly returning to cardiopulmonary bypass, performing an atriotomy or draining blood via the CPB cannulae, if still in situ, allowing rapid reduction in circulating volume and left ventricular preload.

# Mechanical support

Occasionally, despite an optimal circulating volume, epicardial pacing and appropriate inotropic therapy, ventricular function is insufficient to maintain adequate organ perfusion. Under these circumstances mechanical strategies may improve myocardial performance sufficiently to allow separation from CPB. These are discussed briefly here and are dealt with in greater detail in Chapters 9 and 14.

## Chest splinting

Closure of the chest increases intrathoracic pressure and may adversely affect hemodynamics, particularly in right ventricular dysfunction. The chest wound can be left open with the sternum splinted and covered with a dressing, pending closure at a later date when myocardial edema has subsided and cardiac function has improved.

## Intra-aortic balloon counterpulsation

The intra-aortic balloon pump (IABP) consists of a balloon-tipped catheter, usually inserted via the femoral artery to a point in the aorta just distal to the origin of the left subclavian artery. Inflation of the balloon is timed to coincide with the dichrotic notch of the arterial waveform, thus increasing pressure in the aorta during diastole and consequently improving coronary perfusion. The balloon deflates just prior to systole, reducing afterload, left ventricular wall tension and, as a result, myocardial oxygen demand.

IABPs are preferably inserted percutaneously. In high-risk cardiac surgical patients, it is prudent to insert a femoral arterial line prior to CPB, either pre or post induction of anesthesia, when the femoral pulses can be felt. This line can then be used to facilitate percutaneous insertion of IABP if required. The percutaneous approach obviates the need for a surgical "cutdown" and dissection to locate the femoral artery, and importantly avoids the need for surgical removal when the IABP is no longer required.

## Ventricular assist devices (VADs)

Mechanical pumps can be used to assist left, right or biventricular function. These devices are inserted in parallel to one or both ventricles, reducing myocardial work and buying time for the ventricle to recover. VADs should be inserted only when other reasonable options of enhanced cardiac support in the weaning process have been explored.

# Suggested Further Reading

- Gillies M, Bellomo R, Doolan L, Buxton B. Inotropic drug therapy after adult cardiac surgery: a systematic literature review. *Critical Care* 2005; **9**: 266–79.

- Hogue CW, Palin CA, Arrowsmith JE. Cardiopulmonary bypass management and neurological outcomes: an evidence-based appraisal of current practices. *Anesth Analg* 2006; **103**: 21–37.

- Royster RL, Thomas SJ, Davis RF. Termination of cardiopulmonary bypass. In Gravlee GP, Davis RF, Stammers AH, Ungerleider RM, eds. *Cardiopulmonary Bypass: Principles and Practice*, 3rd ed. Philadelphia: Lippincott Williams & Wilkins; 2008: 614–31.

- Shanewise JS, Cheung AT, Aronson S, *et al.* ASE/SCA guidelines for performing a comprehensive intraoperative multiplane transesophageal echocardiography examination: recommendations of the American Society of Echocardiography Council for Intraoperative Echocardiography and the Society of Cardiovascular Anesthesiologists Task Force for Certification in Perioperative Transesophageal Echocardiography. *Anesth Analg* 1999; **89**: 870–84.

# Mechanical circulatory support

Kirsty Dempster and Steven Tsui

The successful introduction of cardiopulmonary bypass in 1953 for closure of an atrial septal defect was an important milestone in the history of circulatory support. Whilst incremental refinements to cardiopulmonary bypass were being made during the ensuing decade, developmental work had already begun with other forms of mechanical circulatory support (MCS). In 1966, a patient who failed to wean from cardiopulmonary bypass due to postcardiotomy shock was successfully bridged-to-recovery with a left ventricular assist device (LVAD). Two years later, a patient with cardiogenic shock was salvaged with an intra-aortic balloon pump. Research on the total artificial heart (TAH) also commenced in the late 1960s.

There are now a wide range of options available for circulatory support (see Table 9.1). This chapter will focus on two of these options: the intra-aortic balloon pump and ventricular assist devices. The decision of whether to proceed to MCS depends on the aetiology of the heart failure and on the likely long-term treatment strategy. Which method of MCS is deployed depends on the acuteness of onset of heart failure, its potential reversibility, its severity and the anticipated duration of support required.

## Intra-aortic balloon counterpulsation

The intra-aortic balloon pump (IABP) is the most commonly used device for circulatory support (see Table 9.2). The balloon catheter has two channels: one for the passage of helium gas used to inflate and deflate the balloon, the other for direct monitoring of intra-aortic blood pressure. It is usually inserted in a retrograde fashion via the femoral artery, with a sheathless insertion technique, causing less obstruction to distal limb perfusion than if the IABP catheter is inserted via a large-bore sheath in the artery. Occasionally, in surgical patients with severe aorto-iliac disease, it is inserted antegrade via the ascending aorta. The IABP catheter is positioned in the descending thoracic aorta, the balloon segment of the catheter lying distal to the origin of the left subclavian artery.

The balloon is rapidly inflated at the end of ventricular systole, just as the aortic valve closes, generating a surge in aortic pressure during ventricular diastole. Just before ventricular systole, the balloon is rapidly deflated, reducing the aortic pressure against which the left ventricle has to eject. The timing of balloon inflation and deflation can be triggered automatically by the patient's ECG or arterial waveform. The combined effects on cardiovascular physiology are listed in Table 9.3.

## Management of the IABP patient

The frequency and degree of balloon augmentation can be controlled via the balloon pump console. The inflation ratio refers to the number of balloon inflations to the number of QRS complexes and can be set at 1:1, 1:2 or 1:3 (see Figure 9.1a–c). The degree of augmentation

**Table 9.1.** Types of mechanical circulatory support

Cardiopulmonary bypass (CPB)

Extracorporeal membrane oxygenation (ECMO)

Intra-aortic balloon pump (IABP)

Ventricular assist devices (VAD)

Total artificial hearts

Cardiac compression devices

Aortic compression devices

**Table 9.2.** Indications for IABP

Ischemic myocardium

- Unstable angina despite maximal medical therapy
- Ischemia-induced ventricular arrhythmia
- Elective support in high-risk percutaneous coronary interventions

Structural complications of acute myocardial infarction

- Ventricular septal defect
- Acute mitral valve regurgitation

Cardiogenic shock

- Post myocardial infarction
- Acute myocarditis
- Acute deterioration of chronic heart failure
- Post cardiotomy
- Acute donor organ failure

can range from 10% to 100%. During normal use, IABP support is initiated with a 1:1 inflation ratio at 100% augmentation. The timing of the inflation/deflation triggers should be checked regularly and adjusted when required to optimize the support provided. To reduce thromboembolic risks associated with an IABP, systemic anticoagulation with heparin infusion is advised, aiming for an activated partial thromboplastin time ratio (APR) of 1.5 to 2.0. Distal limb perfusion must be examined regularly and distal pulses checked either by palpation or with a hand-held Doppler probe.

The effectiveness of IABP augmentation is diminished when there is excessive tachycardia (>120 bpm) or when the cardiac rhythm becomes irregular, e.g., atrial fibrillation (see Figure 9.1e & f). Therefore, inotropic support should be moderated to minimize the occurrence of such rhythm disturbances. Invasive hemodynamic monitoring is indispensable and provides the best assessment of the adequacy of circulatory support. A Swan-Ganz pulmonary artery catheter can provide important information, including left ventricular preload (pulmonary capillary wedge pressure), left ventricular afterload (systemic vascular resistance), right ventricular afterload (pulmonary vascular resistance) and cardiac output as well as providing information on the adequacy of systemic oxygen delivery (mixed venous oxygen saturation). When cardiac function begins to recover, the inotrope dose should be reduced before IABP support is weaned. If cardiac index is maintained above $2.2\,l/minute/m^2$ with acceptable

**Table 9.3.** Beneficial effects of IABP

Balloon deflation during ventricular systole
- Reduces left ventricular afterload
- Reduces peak LV wall stress and LV stroke work
- Decreases myocardial oxygen demand
- Reduces mitral valve regurgitation
- Increases LV ejection

Balloon inflation during ventricular diastole
- Increases coronary perfusion pressure
- Augments coronary blood flow
- Improves myocardial oxygen delivery

Overall effects
- Augments cardiac output
- Reduces pulmonary capillary wedge pressure
- Relieves pulmonary congestion

preload (pulmonary capillary wedge pressure <15 mmHg), attempts can be made to wean the IABP. Firstly, the IABP augmentation can be reduced to 50% for 2–4 hours. The inflation ratio is then progressively reduced from 1:1 to 1:2 for another 2–4 hours and then to 1:3 before the balloon catheter is removed. The IABP must be switched off and the catheter completely deflated just prior to removal. Heparin should be discontinued at the start of IABP weaning so that coagulation is normalized by the time the IABP catheter is removed.

## Complications of IABP use

Major vascular complications can occur in up to 15% of patients treated with an IABP. Femoral insertion of an IABP catheter may not be possible in 5% of patients, because of a tortuous or diseased ilio-femoral system. During insertion, vascular injury can lead to dissection, rupture and hemorrhage. Once in situ, distal limb ischemia can result from thromboembolism or a combination of peripheral vasoconstriction and low cardiac output state. Malpositioning of an IABP catheter may result in obstruction of visceral or renal arteries, making a visual check on catheter position via chest radiography essential.

In the operating room, placement is usually facilitated with the use of transesophageal echocardiography, which is also instrumental in assessing the potential risks of IABP placement from atherosclerotic disease in the thoracic aorta.

Other complications can include infection, thrombocytopenia and rupture of the IABP catheter. Helium is used as the driving gas for IABP inflation because of its high blood solubility, so reducing the risks from gaseous emboli. If the IABP ruptures, blood is seen to track down the gas channel of the balloon driveline. Whenever this is observed, the IABP must be immediately stopped and the catheter removed.

## Ventricular assist devices

Severe heart failure refractory to medical management and IABP support has an appalling prognosis. Inadequate forward perfusion gives rise to end-organ dysfunction and metabolic

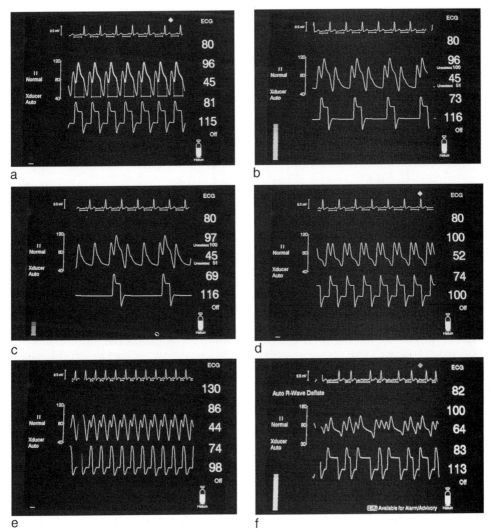

**Figure 9.1** Intra-aortic balloon console tracings. The screen displays ECG at the top, aortic pressure waveform in the center and balloon inflation/deflation at the bottom. (a) Full IABP augmentation with inflation 1:1 and inflation interval highlighted showing correct balloon inflation at the dicrotic notch of the arterial pressure trace. (b & c) Full augmentation with inflation interval 1:2 and 1:3, respectively. (d) Balloon augmentation set at 50%. (e) IABP on full support but showing diminished effectiveness due to tachycardia. (f) Auto R-wave deflate mode for a patient in AF.

acidosis, whilst excessive back-pressure results in pulmonary edema and systemic venous congestion. Ventricular assist devices (VADs) can be used to augment perfusion and relieve congestion, potentially reversing the damaging effects of severe heart failure.

VADs are mechanical blood pumps that can provide either left, right or biventricular support (see Figure 9.2). A left ventricular assist device (LVAD) withdraws oxygenated blood from the left atrium or left ventricle, and returns it to the aorta; a right ventricular assist device (RVAD) draws venous blood from the right atrium or right ventricle, and returns it to the pulmonary artery. In general, it is preferable to cannulate the ventricle for VAD inflow as this provides superior ventricular decompression, avoids ventricular stasis and affords higher VAD flow rates.

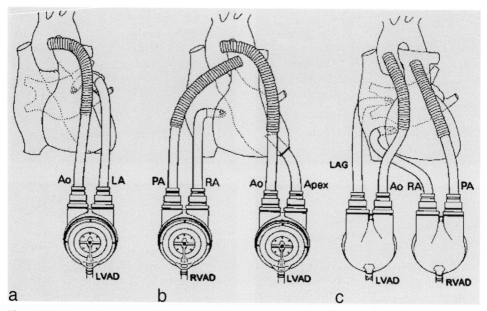

**Figure 9.2** Thoratec Paracorporeal Ventricular Assist Device showing examples of cannulation for LVAD and RVAD. (a) LVAD with cannulation of left atrium (LA) and aorta (Ao). (b) RVAD with cannulation of right atrium (RA) and pulmonary artery (PA) and LVAD with cannulation of left ventricular apex (Apex) and aorta. (c) RVAD with cannulation of right atrium and pulmonary artery and LVAD with cannulation of left atrial inflow (LAG) and aorta.

The output of an LVAD is dependent on adequate right ventricular function to deliver sufficient blood flow across the lungs into the left heart chambers for the LVAD to pump. Likewise, an RVAD can only provide benefit if the native left ventricle can generate enough stroke work to cope with the pulmonary blood flow produced by the RVAD. If both native ventricles are failing, two VADs are required in order to provide biventricular assistance to support the circulation.

In its simplest form, emergency short-term VAD support can be provided by any blood pump (e.g., a Biomedicus centrifugal pump) and a couple of vascular cannulae: one for inflow from the heart to the VAD; the other for outflow return from the VAD to the aorta. In the absence of specialist VAD equipment, such a setup can be lifesaving and maintain the circulation for hours or days.

There is, however, a growing number of pump systems specifically intended for use as a VAD. These systems consist of blood pumps that are less traumatic to the blood components, and have cannulae that are designed to provide more secure attachment to the heart chambers with superior flow characteristics. Temporary VAD systems are intended for short-term circulatory support in the intensive care unit for days or weeks. Long-term VAD systems are designed to provide circulatory support for months or years. Continual improvements in long-term VADs are enabling patients to be discharged from hospital and treated as outpatients, often with a relatively normal quality of life.

The fate of patients receiving a VAD depends on the underlying cause of the cardiac dysfunction and its reversibility. In some cases of postcardiotomy shock and fulminant myocarditis, cardiac function recovers after a period of circulatory support and the VAD can be weaned and removed, a process known as "bridge to recovery." Unfortunately, in the majority of cases of chronic heart failure, e.g., ischemic or dilated cardiomyopathies, the myocardial dysfunction is unlikely to be reversible. Occasionally, a VAD is required for these patients, who are usually already waiting for a heart transplant because of deteriorating cardiac status. Here the VAD is used to buy time for the patient until a suitable donor heart can be found, a process called "bridge to transplant" or BTT. For a selected few patients with advanced heart failure who are not transplant candidates, VAD support can be offered as a permanent implant, a process called "destination therapy" or DT.

## Ventricular assist devices: decision making process

The key decisions of which patient to support with a VAD, when to insert a VAD, whether the patient requires LVAD alone or BiVAD and which VAD system to use are often difficult ones to make. They are influenced by a number of factors including patient comorbidities, transplant waiting times, resource availability, institutional experience and device availability. In general, patients who are considered for VAD support can be divided into the following four categories (see Table 9.4).

- **Group I** – This consists of transplant-eligible patients with precarious hemodynamics who are managed on the intensive care unit. They are the most challenging group of patients to make a decision on because a rush to implant a VAD too early may "deny" them a more straightforward course of heart transplantation without mechanical bridging, whereas waiting too long for a donor heart may result in end-organ failure or, worse still, cardiac arrest and death. In these cases, it is important to monitor the trends in hemodynamics as well as inotrope requirements. Adequacy of end-organ function is best assessed by monitoring hourly urine output, arterial oxygenation, prothrombin time and acid–base balance. In the United Kingdom, where the median waiting time for an "urgent" donor heart is 2 or 3 weeks, most of these patients can be transplanted without needing VAD support. In other countries, where the minimum waiting time for an "urgent" heart runs into many months, most of these patients are treated with a VAD. Ventricular tachy-arrhythmia is an ominous sign and should prompt an earlier decision for VAD insertion. Since the "bridging" period to a transplant can range from months to sometimes over a year, these patients should be implanted with a long-term VAD so that they can be discharged home. Currently, there are several wearable or portable VAD systems that allow patients independent mobility during VAD support with reasonable quality of life. Patients in this category have an 80–90% chance of being successfully bridged to a heart transplant if treated with a VAD.

**Table 9.4.** Categories of patients considered for VAD insertion

| Group | Description |
|---|---|
| I Precarious | Severe heart failure with borderline hemodynamics requiring inotropic therapy +/– IABP |
| II Decompensated | Untransplantable due to acute end-organ failure or chronically raised pulmonary vascular resistance (>6 Wood units) |
| III Failure to wean from CPB | Postcardiotomy shock or acute donor organ failure after heart transplant |
| IV Salvage | Cardiac arrest refractory to CPR |

- **Group II** – This consists of patients who are transplant candidates except for one or more serious, but potentially reversible, complications of advanced heart failure, e.g., acute end-organ failure or pulmonary hypertension. Unless such complication(s) can be reversed, these patients are not transplantable and they will invariably die from their heart failure. Acute end-organ failure secondary to a low cardiac output state sometimes recovers when the systemic circulation is mechanically augmented; elevated pulmonary vascular resistance due to left ventricular failure and pulmonary venous congestion often decreases with mechanical unloading of the left ventricle. This category of patients are sick and those who survive the surgery of VAD implant often require weeks or months of VAD support to reverse their end-organ failure before they are acceptable for a heart transplant. It is therefore most appropriate to consider a long-term VAD system in these cases. Operative risks are higher in this decompensated group and only 60–70% of them will survive to a heart transplant.
- **Group III** – This consists of patients who could not be weaned from cardiopulmonary bypass despite maximal inotropic therapy and IABP support. This includes patients with postcardiotomy shock and those with acute donor organ failure following heart transplantation. In the absence of contraindications (see Table 9.5), a short-term VAD may be considered to enable weaning from CPB. Alternatively, a veno-arterial ECMO circuit may be used to support the circulation. Injured hearts that are likely to recover tend to do so within 5–7 days. If weaning from MCS cannot be accomplished after this period because of ongoing poor ventricular function, a decision has to be made between device removal and death, or continued support and bridging to transplantation (or re-transplantation). Occasionally, it may be felt appropriate to switch over to a long-term device to wait for a suitable donor heart. Overall survival rate for the postcardiotomy group is poor at 30–40%.
- **Group IV** – This consists of patients with catastrophic heart failure/cardiac arrest who have been put onto CPB or ECMO for resuscitation under cardiopulmonary resuscitation (CPR) conditions. These patients tend to be young, previously fit and would normally be good candidates for heart transplantation. The main uncertainty that exists concerns the patient's neurological status following a period of cardiopulmonary resuscitation. Again, a short-term VAD or veno-arterial ECMO may be used to support

**Table 9.5.** Contraindications to use of VADs postcardiotomy

| |
|---|
| Age >65 years |
| Uncontrollable bleeding |
| Intractable metabolic acidosis |
| Other comorbidities |
| · Pre-existing neurological impairment |
| · Severe cerebral vascular disease |
| · Severe peripheral vascular disease |
| · Advanced chronic pulmonary disease |
| · Chronic renal failure |
| · Chronic liver disease |
| · Recent malignancy |

the circulation until neurological assessment can be conducted. Severe neurological injury usually becomes obvious within 48 hours of circulatory support, permitting withdrawal of treatment. Otherwise, consideration may have to be given to bridging to transplantation or switching to a longer term device.

# Types of ventricular assist devices

Technical developments in mechanical circulatory support have progressed rapidly over the last 10 years. There is now a large range of systems available for clinical use. These can be classified into temporary systems and long-term systems. Within each group, they can be subdivided into volume displacement devices (pulsatile devices) and continuous flow devices (see Table 9.6). There has been much debate over pulsatile versus continuous flow pumps, but recent studies have shown no differences in end-organ function and patient survival between the two types of devices. A full description of all available devices is beyond the scope of this book. A few selected examples of commonly available VADs that are in clinical use are briefly described below.

**Table 9.6.** Classification and examples of VAD systems

A. Temporary devices:
- Volume displacement
  - Abiomed BVS 5000 and AB5000
  - Medos
- Continuous flow
  - Impella
  - CardiacAssist TandemHeart
  - Levitronix CentriMag*

B. Longer term devices:
- Volume displacement
  - Abiomed AB5000
  - Berlin Excor
  - Thoratec HeartMate XVE
  - Novacor
  - Thoratec PVAD
  - Thoratec IVAD
- Continuous flow
  - Micromed DeBakey
  - Jarvik 2000 Flowmaker
  - Thoratec HeartMate II
  - Berlin Incor*
  - Ventracor VentrAssist*
  - Terumo Duraheart*
  - HeartWare HVAD*

* The latest bearing-less designs.

## Levitronix CentriMag

The Levitronix CentriMag is a continuous flow extracorporeal system comprising a single-use polycarbonate centrifugal pump, a motor and a primary drive console (see Figures 9.3 and 9.4). It is intended for short-term left, right or biventricular support of up to 30 days' duration. Compared to other short-term devices, the Levitronix CentriMag is unique in that it is designed to operate without mechanical bearings or seals, which are components known to contribute to hemolysis and thrombus formation. The magnetically suspended impeller achieves rotation with no friction or wear at speeds of 1500–5500 rpm, providing flow rates of up to 9.9 l/minute in vitro. In vivo, flows of 4.0–5.0 l/minute are often observed.

The inflow and outflow cannulae can be rapidly inserted into the heart and great vessels with or without cardiopulmonary bypass (see Figure 9.5). Other clinical equipment such as a membrane oxygenator or hemofilter can be spliced into the system. Although patients supported with the CentriMag are kept on the intensive care unit, they can be allowed to move around the bed space and can undergo physiotherapy. Because of its simplicity and versatility, the CentriMag is becoming rapidly adopted by many cardiothoracic centers.

## Thoratec PVAD and IVAD

The Thoratec system was originally designed as a pulsatile paracorporeal ventricular assist device (PVAD), which can be used for either left, right or biventricular support (see Figure 9.2). The pump unit consists of a polyurethane blood sac and Bjork-Shiley monostrut inflow and outflow mechanical valves, inside a rigid polysulfone case (see Figure 9.6). A range of inflow cannulae allow either left or right atrial or ventricular cannulation. The outflow cannula can be attached to the ascending aorta or the pulmonary artery. The inflow and outflow cannulae are passed across the abdominal wall and the pump unit rests in front of the abdomen. The VAD is connected to an external pneumatic drive console via a gas line and can provide pulsatile support of up to 6.5 l/minute.

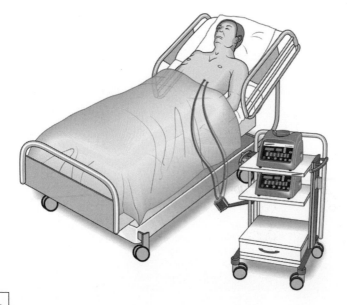

**Figure 9.3** Levitronix CentriMag Primary Console and patient.

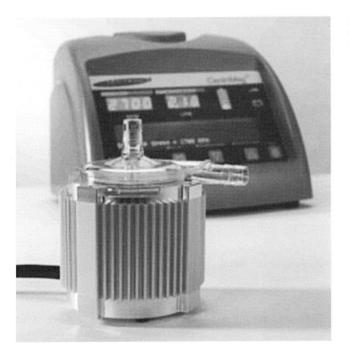

**Figure 9.4** Levitronix CentriMag Pump, Motor and Primary Drive Console.

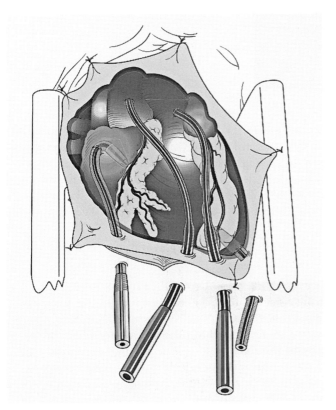

**Figure 9.5** Example of BiVAD cannulation with the LVAD inflow cannula in the LV apex and the outflow cannula returning blood to the ascending aorta. The RVAD inflow cannula takes blood from the right atrium with the outflow cannula returning blood to the pulmonary artery. The cannulae are tunneled through the skin to allow for chest closure.

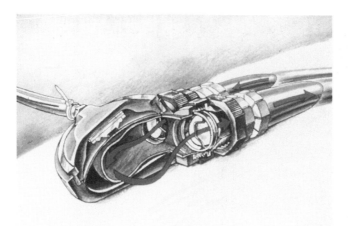

**Figure 9.6** The cutaway view shows the internal components of the PVAD. Blood passes from a percutaneous inflow cannula, through a mechanical tilting disc valve that maintains unidirectional flow, and into the polyurethane blood sac. On exertion of drive pressure, blood is forced out of the VAD through another mechanical valve and into the outflow cannula, to return to the patient.

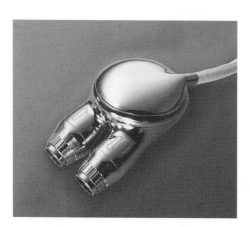

**Figure 9.7** Thoratec IVAD with its streamlined titanium housing and velour-coated percutaneous lead.

More recently, Thoratec has taken the PVAD design and adapted it into an implantable ventricular assist device (IVAD) by substituting the polysulfone case with a more streamlined titanium housing (see Figure 9.7). Along the lines of the PVAD, the Thoratec IVAD can be used as left or right ventricular support as well as biventricular support using two complete units. This implantable version makes the system much more acceptable for the patients and their carers (see Figure 9.8) and it is currently the only implantable VAD that can provide support for either ventricle.

## HeartMate II

The HeartMate II is a high-speed, axial flow blood pump. It is a compact device weighing 400 g and measuring approximately 4 cm in diameter and 6 cm long and, as such, it may be suitable for a wider range of patients, including small adults and children.

The internal pump surfaces are a smooth, polished titanium. A rotor within the pump contains a magnet and is rotated by the electromotive force generated by the integral magnetic motor (see Figure 9.9). The rotor spins on blood-lubricated ceramic bearings, and propels the blood from the inflow cannula sited in the LV apex to the ascending aorta. The pump speed can vary from 6000 to 15 000 rpm, providing blood flow of up to 10 l/minute.

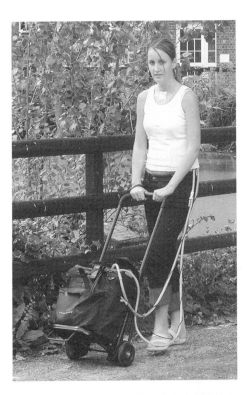

**Figure 9.8** Patient support with two IVADs mobilizing with the Thoratec portable TLC-II driver.

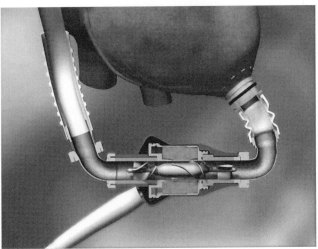

**Figure 9.9** Cutaway view of HeartMate II showing inflow cannula in the left ventricle, rotor, magnetic motor and ceramic bearings, and outflow towards ascending aorta.

The pump can run in two operating modes: fixed speed and auto-speed. In fixed-speed mode, the device operates at a constant speed, which can be adjusted via the system monitor. In the auto-speed mode, the pump speed varies in response to different levels of patient or cardiac activity.

External equipment includes a system controller, power base unit, system monitor, rechargeable batteries and battery clips. The system controller continuously monitors and controls the implanted pump and shows information regarding alarm conditions.

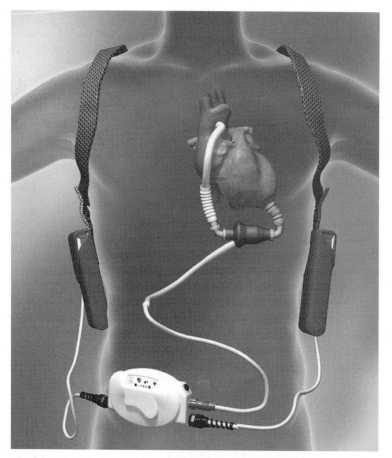

**Figure 9.10** Diagram of the configuration of the HeartMate II showing implanted pump, percutaneous lead, external system controller and batteries.

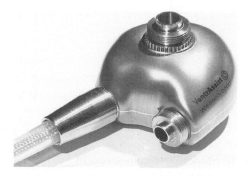

**Figure 9.11** Ventracor VentrAssist.

The power base unit serves as a battery charger and an interface between the system monitor and the implanted pump. The 20-foot power cable allows the system to be operated by AC power. Alternatively, patients can connect to batteries, which permits the system to be operated tether-free for 3–5 hours (see Figure 9.10).

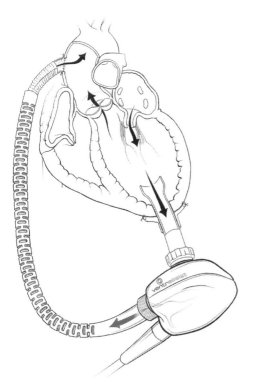

**Figure 9.12** Inflow to the VentrAssist is from the LV apex and outflow to the ascending aorta. The percutaneous driveline is tunneled out through the skin. Despite being a continuous flow device, some pulsatility of flow may be detectable with native ventricular contractions.

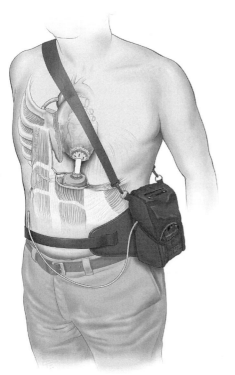

**Figure 9.13** Ventracor's compact backpack containing controller and batteries.

## Ventracor VentrAssist

The VentrAssist is one of the latest generations of longer term LVADs consisting of a small implantable titanium centrifugal pump (see Figures 9.11, 9.12, 9.13), percutaneous driveline, portable controller and rechargeable battery packs. When activated, the impeller is hydrodynamically suspended on a thin film of blood and requires no conventional bearing. By eliminating the potential for mechanical wear and tear, these pumps are designed for maximum durability. Continuous flow devices tend to be smaller in size than pulsatile devices, and are quiet in operation, making them less intrusive to live with. It is hoped that these devices can provide long-term circulatory support with lower morbidity and mortality.

# VAD patient management

## Preoperative management

Patients requiring a VAD implant are probably amongst the sickest patients to undergo cardiac surgery. They have severe heart failure and are either in impending or established end-organ failure. A low cardiac output state coupled with systemic venous congestion result in compromised organ perfusion. The kidneys become refractory to diuretic therapy and hepatic dysfunction manifests as coagulation abnormalities. The lungs are stiff from pulmonary congestion, increasing the work of breathing, and many patients are grossly fluid overloaded.

If the stability of the patient permits, a period of *preoperative* optimization in the ICU prior to VAD implant can be highly beneficial. Inotropic therapy should be rationalized to reduce the risk of arrhythmias and a period of IABP support helps augment end-organ perfusion. Furthermore, the IABP reduces left atrial pressure, thereby reducing the work of the right ventricle indirectly. Low-dose vitamin K can normalize an elevated prothrombin time, which in turn reduces the risk of perioperative hemorrhage.

Continuous veno-venous hemofiltration (CVVH) is the most expeditious way of reducing excessive intravascular volume and total body water content. Patients with chronic heart failure with CVP >20 mmHg are often grossly edematous. The aim is to normalize the preload and bring the CVP towards 10–12 mmHg. In practice, CVVH can be used to give a negative balance of 600–1000 ml per hour until the target CVP is reached. In these patients, it is not uncommon to remove 7–10 l of fluid in the first 24 hours of CVVH. As the venous pressure begins to normalize, excessive fluid from the third spaces also returns to the intravascular compartment and peripheral edema resolves. Finally, by normalizing an elevated preload, the overstretched ventricles and atrio-ventricular valves are allowed to return to more physiological dimensions, often resulting in improvements in function of the atrio-ventricular valves.

The combined use of IABP and CVVH support in fluid overloaded patients in a low cardiac output state often results in augmentation of cardiac output and tissue oxygen delivery, as measured by improvements in mixed venous oxygen saturations.

## Perioperative management

The perioperative strategy should be aimed at minimizing further insult to these sick patients during VAD implantation, targeting those areas that are known to result in serious morbidities and mortality. Perhaps the most unpredictable and dangerous complication following LVAD implantation is right ventricular failure. It is therefore imperative to pay particular

**Table 9.7.** Factors contributing to right ventricular failure following LVAD

Right ventricular dysfunction
- Right ventricular ischemia
- Deviation of the interventricular septum to the left
- Air embolism into the right coronary artery
- Right ventricular volume overload and overdistension

Functional regurgitation of tricuspid valve

Elevated pulmonary vascular resistance
- Atelectasis
- Metabolic acidosis
- Pulmonary vasospasm

**Table 9.8.** Perioperative LVAD patient management

Broad-spectrum prophylactic antibiotics and antifungal agents

Trans-esophageal echocardiography
- Confirm aortic valve competence
- Exclude patent foramen ovale and ASD
- Confirm de-airing
- Check LVAD cannula position
- Confirm decompression of LA and LV during LVAD support
- Monitor right ventricular and tricuspid valve function when weaning from CPB

Normothermic cardiopulmonary bypass

Continuous ventilation of the lungs with nitric oxide at 10 ppm

Filtration on CPB and maintain
- Hb >10 g/dl
- Base excess ± 2 mEq

No aortic cross-clamp during VAD cannulae implant

Pericardial $CO_2$

Dopamine infusion at 5 μg/kg/minute or appropriate inotropic support for right ventricle

Vasopressin infusion for SVR

attention to factors that might contribute to this complication (see Table 9.7). The other commonly encountered problem is early postoperative hemorrhage.

The VAD implant procedure should be covered by broad-spectrum prophylactic antibiotics and antifungal agents. Trans-esophageal echocardiography (TOE) is used to confirm aortic valve competence and exclude the presence of a patent foramen ovale or an atrial septal defect. If present, they require surgical closure at the time of VAD implant, in order to prevent a right to left shunt following decompression of the left-sided chambers with an LVAD. The lungs can be kept ventilated throughout the bypass period with the addition of nitric oxide at 10 parts per million (ppm) to minimize atelectasis and pulmonary vasoconstriction, respectively. We advocate normothermic cardiopulmonary bypass using hemofiltration (ultrafiltration) to help maintain hemoglobin >10 g/dl and base excess within ±2 mEq/l. The VAD cannulae are implanted into a beating heart, avoiding aortic cross-clamping and cardiac ischemia. The pericardial space is flooded with carbon dioxide so that gas bubbles entrained into cardiac chambers can dissolve more readily. The right ventricle is supported with an infusion of dopamine at 5 μg/kg/minute. The heart rate is optimized with temporary pacing at 90–100 bpm. Systemic vascular resistance is maintained between 800 and 1000 dyn.s/cm$^5$ using an infusion of vasopressin or with an alpha-agonist. Thorough de-airing of the heart is confirmed with TOE before finally attempting to wean from bypass.

The perioperative management strategy is summarized in Table 9.8.

## Weaning from CPB with VAD support

In order to wean from CPB, the heart is filled to a CVP of 8–10 mmHg. Once TOE confirms that the left-sided cardiac chambers are sufficiently filled, the LVAD is initiated at the lowest possible setting. As the LVAD flow rate increases, CPB is gradually reduced, taking care not to overdistend the right ventricle. It is sometimes necessary to supplement the LVAD output with CPB flows of 1–2 l/minute for the first 20–30 minutes before complete weaning. TOE is used to confirm satisfactory LVAD cannula position and left heart decompression. TOE is particularly useful in determining the adequacy of LV filling and monitoring the response of the RV as CPB support is weaned; collapse of the LV wall around the LVAD cannula, or septal distortion, are readily observed by TOE and indicate that the balance between the set LVAD flow rate and cardiac filling needs to be addressed and that RV function may need to be further optimized.

If LVAD flows of 2.2 l/minute/m$^2$ cannot be achieved with CVP <15 mmHg, adequacy of tissue perfusion should be assessed with mixed venous oxygen saturation measurement ($S_vO_2$). Not infrequently, patients suffering from chronic heart failure are already accustomed to a low cardiac output state and a cardiac index of 1.8 l/minute/m$^2$ may be quite acceptable provided that the $S_vO_2$ is satisfactory (> preimplant $S_vO_2$). Otherwise additional measures to augment LVAD flows have to be considered.

As mentioned earlier, the output of an LVAD is dependent upon adequate right ventricular function to deliver enough blood flow across the lungs to the left-sided cardiac chambers and LVAD inflow. If LVAD flows are inadequate and the left heart appears empty on TOE despite a full right heart, this is either due to right ventricular failure, elevated pulmonary artery resistance or a combination of both. These can either be treated with low-dose infusions of adrenaline and a phosphodiesterase inhibitor or with inhaled iloprost, respectively. However, unless LVAD flows improve readily, CPB should be reinstituted early to avoid development of metabolic acidosis. Under these circumstances, the early addition of a RVAD is advisable to provide bi-ventricular support.

## Postoperative management of VAD patients

At the end of the VAD implant, careful hemostasis is crucial in order to minimize hemorrhage. An effective closed drainage system is essential in preventing mediastinal and pump pocket collections. Some surgeons close the pericardial sac or place a surgical membrane between the sternum and the mediastinum to facilitate subsequent re-sternotomy and re-entry. The percutaneous cannulae or driveline must be secured externally in order to minimize movement and trauma to the exit site(s). This is the best way to encourage tissue healing onto the driveline and minimize exit site infections.

Once returned to the intensive care unit, VAD patients must be closely monitored for early complications (see Table 9.9). Antibiotic prophylaxis is continued for 48 hours. Coagulation defects should be corrected without waiting for signs of bleeding. Right ventricular (RV) function often remains precarious in the first few days following LVAD implantation. RV failure can be precipitated by excessive LVAD flow rate and/or elevated pulmonary vascular resistance (PVR). Therefore, it is prudent to limit the LVAD flow rate in the first few days in order to avoid overwhelming the RV or shifting the ventricular septum to the left and distorting RV dynamics. Furthermore, it is essential to avoid factors that may precipitate increases in PVR, e.g., hypoxia and acidosis.

Anticoagulation is usually omitted in the first 24 hours and is only introduced when the patient has stopped bleeding (<30 ml/hour for 3 consecutive hours). Most institutions commence with an infusion of unfractionated heparin and this is continued for 5–7 days before warfarin is commenced. The actual anticoagulation/antiplatelet regimen is device specific and also unit specific.

Rising right atrial pressure coupled with a fall in pump flow rate are signs of tamponade or impending RV failure. The latter can be confirmed with TOE, which demonstrates full right-sided cardiac chambers with empty left-sided chambers. The atrial and ventricular septa are seen to bulge towards the left and these are often accompanied by tricuspid valve regurgitation. Under these circumstances, it is important not to increase the preload further with fluid transfusions. Immediate treatment consists of a combination of inotropic support for the RV and pulmonary vasodilators. These may include adrenaline (up to 0.1 µg/kg/minute), enoximone (5 µg/kg/minute), nitric oxide (up to 20 parts per million) and/or nebulized iloprost (9.9 µg 3 hourly). If the situation does not respond readily to these measures, early consideration should be given to the addition of an RVAD.

## Long-term care

Long-term support of a VAD patient relies on a multidisciplinary approach. Dieticians are involved from the preoperative period to ensure that nutrition is optimized. Most patients would have been immobile for a long period of time and will require intensive physiotherapy to facilitate their physical rehabilitation postoperatively. Anticoagulation therapy has to be closely monitored to reduce the risk of thromboembolic and hemorrhagic complications. The patient will need to be taught how to care for their driveline exit site to minimize the risk of

**Table 9.9.** Common complications of VAD support

| |
| --- |
| Perioperative hemorrhage |
| Right ventricular failure |
| Cerebral vascular events |
| · Metabolic |
| · Embolic |
| · Hemorrhagic |
| Infection |
| Hemolysis |
| Thromboembolism |
| Mechanical pump failure |

infection. The patient will also need to be trained in all aspects of operating and maintaining their VAD system, allowing them the freedom and independence to leave the hospital and return to a normal life.

## Suggested Further Reading

- Frazier OH, Kirklin J *Mechanical Circulatory Support. ISHLT Monograph Series.* New York: Elsevier; 2006.

- Goldstein D, Oz MC. *Cardiac Assist Devices.* London: Blackwell Publishing Ltd; 2002.

- Rose E, Gelijns AC, Moskowitz AJ, *et al.* Long-term use of a left ventricular assist device for end-stage heart failure. *New Engl J Med* 2001; **345**(20): 1435–43 (rematch trial).

- Samuels L, Narula J. Ventricular assist devices and the artificial heart. *Cardiol Clin* 2003; **21**(1).

- Tsui S, Parameshwar J. Mechanical circulatory support. *Core Topics Cardiothorac Critl Care* 2008: 157–66.

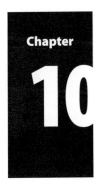

# Chapter 10

# Deep hypothermic circulatory arrest

Joe Arrowsmith and Charles W. Hogue

The majority of cardiac surgical procedures are accomplished using cardioplegia-induced cardiac arrest with cardiopulmonary bypass (CPB) to maintain perfusion to other organs. However, in certain situations, the nature of the surgical procedure or the pathology of the underlying condition necessitates complete cessation of blood flow. For example, safe removal of large tumors encroaching on vascular structures requires provision of a bloodless field to enable dissection, or operations on the aorta itself may preclude application of a cross-clamp because of the pathological anatomy. Preservation of organ function during the period of total circulatory arrest can be aided by reducing the core temperature of the body. The technique of core cooling combined with cessation of blood flow is termed "deep hypothermic circulatory arrest" (DHCA).

DHCA provides excellent operating conditions – albeit of limited duration – whilst ameliorating the major adverse consequences of organ ischemia. During DHCA the brain is the organ most vulnerable to injury, but may be protected if cooled to reduce its metabolic activity, and hence oxygen requirements, before and during the period of arrest. Similarly, preservation of the function of other organs less susceptible to ischemic damage may be afforded by core cooling. DHCA owes its existence to two overlapping eras; a brief period in the early 1950s when hypothermia was used as the sole method for organ protection during surgery and the current epoch of CPB heralded by Gibbon in 1953. Subsequent modifications to the basic technique have extended both the duration of "safe" circulatory arrest and the range of surgical indications.

## Historical roots

In pioneering work during the 1940s and early 1950s, Bigelow demonstrated that a reduction in body temperature to 30°C increased the period of "safe" cerebral ischemia from 3 to 10 minutes – time enough for expeditious intracardiac surgery. Hypothermic inflow occlusion in cardiac surgery was first successfully achieved using cold rubber blankets for surface cooling. The use of an iced water bath for cooling proved more practical and was adopted by others with considerable success, notably in London by Holmes Sellors. The types of procedures that could be undertaken during inflow occlusion, however, were limited to atrial septal defect repair, valvotomy and valvectomy. More profound degrees of hypothermia were later described. Despite spectacular successes, the incidence of death and complications such as hypothermia-induced ventricular fibrillation, hemorrhage, myocardial failure and neurological injury were high by today's standards.

Although CPB-induced hypothermia and DHCA in the management of aortic arch pathology had been described in the 1960s, it was Griepp, in 1975, who demonstrated that the technique offered a relatively simple and safe approach for aortic arch surgery. DHCA, either alone or in combination with other strategies, has remained the mainstay of brain protection

*Cardiopulmonary Bypass*, ed. S. Ghosh, F. Falter and D. J. Cook. Published by Cambridge University Press.
© Cambridge University Press 2009.

**Table 10.1.** Applications of deep hypothermic circulatory arrest

| | |
|---|---|
| Cardiothoracic surgery | Thoracic aortic surgery |
| | Pulmonary (thrombo) endarterectomy |
| | Complex pediatric reconstructions |
| Neurosurgery | Basilar artery aneurysm surgery |
| | Cerebral tumor resection |
| | Intracranial arterio-venous malformation resection |
| Other | Caval mass resection (e.g., renal cell carcinoma) |

during aortic surgery. In addition to being used to facilitate pulmonary vascular surgery and the repair of congenital cardiac lesions, DHCA may also be used in both neurosurgery and urological surgery (see Table 10.1).

# Pathophysiology of hypothermia

In animals that maintain body temperature in a tight range, homeotherms, thermoregulation occurs as a result of the dynamic balance between heat production (thermogenesis) and heat loss. Stimulation of cutaneous cold receptors and temperature-sensitive neurons in the hypothalamus activate vasoconstrictive, endocrine, adaptive behavioral and shivering mechanisms to maintain core temperature. Hypothermia, defined as a core temperature <35°C, occurs when heat losses overwhelm thermoregulatory mechanisms (e.g., during cold immersion) or when thermoregulation is impaired by pathological conditions (e.g., stroke, trauma, endocrinopathy, sepsis, autonomic neuropathy, uremia) or drugs (e.g., anesthetic agents, barbiturates, benzodiazepines, phenothiazines, ethanol). Thanks to the early work of Rosomoff and Currie (Rosomoff 1956), and experience gained from managing accidental hypothermia, the physiological effects of hypothermia are well known (see Table 10.2). An understanding of both normal physiological and pathological responses is essential when using deliberate or therapeutic hypothermia.

# Practical considerations

Preoperative assessment is similar to that for any other major cardiac surgical procedure. Because DHCA is commonly used in emergent, life-saving procedures it may not be possible to undertake the usual battery of "routine" preoperative investigations. The presence of significant comorbidities (e.g., coronary artery disease, cerebrovascular disease, renal insufficiency, diabetes mellitus) should be anticipated on the basis of the clinical history and physical examination.

## Anesthesia

Standard arterial, central venous and peripheral venous access is required in all cases. In anticipation of division of the innominate vein to improve surgical access, venous cannulae should be sited in the right arm or in the femoral vein. Cannulation of the right radial artery and a femoral artery permits arterial pressure monitoring both proximal and distal to the aortic arch. Cannulation of a femoral artery also serves as an anatomical marker for the surgeon should an intra-aortic balloon pump be required on separation from CPB. Whilst not considered mandatory, pulmonary artery catheterization may aid

**Table 10.2.** The pathophysiology of hypothermia

| | Mild 33–35°C | Moderate 28–33°C | Severe <28°C |
|---|---|---|---|
| Neurological | Confusion<br>Amnesia<br>Apathy<br>Impaired judgment | Depressed consciousness | Pupillary dilatation<br>Coma<br>Loss of autoregulation |
| Neuromuscular | Shivering<br>Ataxia<br>Dysarthria | Muscle and joint stiffening | Muscle rigor |
| Cardiovascular | Tachycardia<br>Vasoconstriction<br>Increased BP, CO | Bradycardia<br>Increased SVR<br>Decreased cardiac output<br>ECG changes:<br>– J (Osborn) waves<br>– QRS broadening<br>– ST elevation/depression<br>– T wave inversion<br>– AV block<br>– QT prolongation | Severe bradycardia Asystole<br>Ventricular fibrillation |
| Respiratory | Tachypnea<br>Left-shift $HbO_2$ curve | Bradypnea<br>Bronchospasm<br>Bronchorrhea | Lactic acidosis<br>Right-shift $HbO_2$ curve |
| Renal/metabolic | Antidiuretic hormone resistance<br>Cold-induced diuresis | Reduced glomerular filtration rate<br>Reduced $H^+$ and glucose reabsorption | Metabolic acidosis |
| Hematology | Increased blood viscosity and hemoconcentration (2% increase in hemacrit/°C) | | |
| | Coagulopathy – inhibition of intrinsic/extrinsic pathway enzymes, platelet activation, thrombocytopenia (liver sequestration) | | |
| | Leukocyte depletion, impaired neutrophil function and bacterial phagocytosis | | |
| Gastrointestinal | | Reduced motility<br>Acute pancreatitis | Ileus<br>Gastric ulcers<br>Hepatic dysfunction |

management immediately post-CPB and in the early postoperative period. Where available, and in the absence of contraindications, transesophageal echocardiography (TOE) may be used to assess aortic valvular function, monitor cardiac function and assist with cardiac de-airing.

Accurate temperature monitoring – at two or more sites – is crucial. Nasopharyngeal or tympanic membrane temperature monitoring provides an indication of brain temperature, whereas rectal or bladder temperature monitoring provides an indication of body core temperature. Whilst these devices are accurate at *steady-state* it should be borne in mind that, during both cooling and warming, thermal gradients may be generated in tissues and monitored temperature may lag behind actual tissue temperature by 2–5°C.

The choice of anesthetic drugs is largely a matter of personal and institutional preference. In theory, using propofol and opioid-based anesthesia in preference to volatile anesthetic agents, reduces cerebral metabolism without uncoupling flow–metabolism relationships. The impact of hypothermia on drug metabolism and elimination should be considered and drug infusion rates adjusted accordingly.

The long duration of surgery with DHCA mandates careful attention to prevent pressure sores and inadvertent damage to the eyes, nerve plexuses, peripheral nerves and pressure points. Cannulation sites, three-way taps, monitoring lines, the endotracheal tube connector and TOE probe should be padded to prevent pressure necrosis of the skin.

All measures should be taken to facilitate re-warming and prevent "after-drop" hypothermia following the termination of CPB. The use of a heated mattress, sterile forced-air blanket and intravenous fluid warmer should be considered in all cases.

## Surgical considerations

In some cases, such as acute type A aortic dissection, femoral or right axillary arterial cannulation may initially be necessary together with femoral venous cannulation to establish CPB. Femoro-femoral or axillo-femoral CPB permits systemic cooling prior to sternotomy and affords a degree of organ protection should chest-opening be accompanied by inadvertent damage to the aorta, or heart, and exsanguination. After completion of the aortic repair, placement of the arterial line directly into the prosthetic graft restores antegrade flow. Cannulation of the mid or distal aortic arch may be required in cases of degenerative aortic aneurysm to reduce the risk of atheroembolism associated with retrograde flow via femoral arterial cannulation.

The choice of venous drainage site and cannula is largely dictated by surgical preference and the degree of access necessary. For example, bicaval cannulation is required if retrograde cerebral perfusion (RCP) is to be used with reversal of blood flow in the superior vena cava. If antegrade cerebral perfusion is to be used with selective arterial cannulation of the carotid arterial circulation then adequate cerebral venous drainage must be ensured, again using bicaval cannulation, to optimize cerebral perfusion pressure and prevent cerebral edema. Alternatively, selective antegrade cerebral perfusion may be obtained by arterial inflow into the right subclavian artery. This potentially allows near continuous low flow to at least the right cerebral hemisphere by the brachiocephalic artery. This technique simplifies the surgical field by elimination of carotid cannulation for antegrade perfusion and may reduce risk of embolism or vessel injury. Removal of a renal tumor from the inferior vena cava requires the use of a right atrial basket – in preference to a caval or two-stage cannula – to permit full visualization of the cava and to prevent dislodged fragments of tumor from becoming impacted in the pulmonary circulation.

The use of DHCA during surgery of the distal aorta via left thoractomy presents several problems. Access to the proximal aorta is limited and femoral arterial cannulation may be required initially. Access to the right atrium typically requires an extensive thoracotomy that traverses the sternum. Alternatively, venous drainage may be achieved using pulmonary artery cannulation or a long femoral cannula advanced into the right atrium.

# Extracorporeal circulation

The nature of DHCA sometimes requires modifications to be made to the standard extracorporeal circuit including:

- infusion bags for the storage of heparinized blood during hemodilution (see below);
- use of a centrifugal pump – in preference to a roller pump – which may reduce damage to the cellular components of the circulation and reduce hemolysis;
- incorporation of a hemofilter to control acidosis and hyperkalemia and enable hemoconcentration during re-warming;
- incorporation of a leukocyte-depleting arterial line filter (see below);
- selection of a cardiotomy reservoir of sufficient capacity to accommodate the circulating volume during exsanguination immediately before DHCA;
- arterio-venous bypass and accessory arterial lines – to permit retrograde or selective antegrade cerebral perfusion (see below);
- an efficient heat exchanger. Assuming that human tissue has an average specific heat capacity of 3.5 kJ/kg/°C (0.83 kcal/kg/°C), the energy required to warm a 70 kg adult from 20°C to 37°C is at least 4.2 MJ (1000 kcal) – the equivalent of the energy required to raise the temperature of 12.5 l water from 20°C to 100°C; and
- the use of heparin-bonded circuits is advocated in cases requiring prolonged CPB, although there is no conclusive evidence of benefit.

## Cooling

Following anticoagulation, CPB is instituted with a constant flow rate of 2.4 l/minute/m² and cooling immediately commenced with a water bath to a blood temperature gradient of <10°C. Vasoconstrictors (e.g., phenylephrine, metaraminol) or vasodilators (e.g., glyceryl trinitrate, nitroprusside) are used to ensure a mean arterial pressure of 50–60 mmHg. As much of the planned procedure as possible is carried out *during* the cooling phase *prior* to DHCA, in order to minimize the duration of circulatory arrest.

Cooling continues until brain (e.g., nasopharyngeal) and core body (e.g., bladder) temperatures have equilibrated at the target temperature for 10–15 minutes. In some centers, continuous monitoring of the EEG, evoked potentials or jugular venous saturation is used as a guide to the adequacy of cerebral cooling.

## Circulatory arrest

As stated earlier, every effort should be made to reduce the period of ischemia. For this reason preparation of any prosthetic grafts and as much surgical dissection as possible should be undertaken during the period of cooling. The operating table is then placed in a slightly head-down (Trendelenberg) position, the pump stopped, intravenous infusions stopped and the patient partially exsanguinated into the venous reservoir. Once isolated from the patient, blood within the extracorporeal circuit is recirculated via a connection between the arterial and venous lines in order to prevent stagnation and clotting. The surgical repair proceeds with heed to the duration of circulatory arrest.

## Safe duration of DHCA

Determining the duration of DHCA that any particular patient will tolerate without sustaining disabling neurological injury remains, at best, an inexact science. Current practice makes

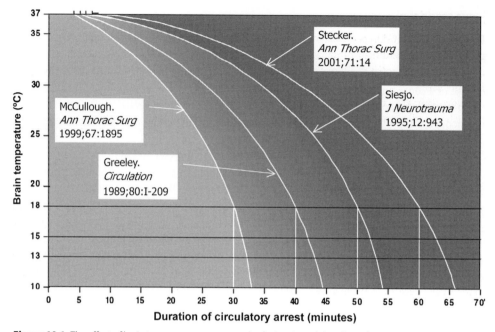

**Figure 10.1** The effect of brain temperature on reported safe duration of deep hypothermic circulatory arrest duration.

it difficult to separate the neurological risks of prolonged CPB, reperfusion and re-warming – all unavoidable consequences of DHCA – from those of DHCA alone. The incidence of neurological injury rises sharply when DHCA exceeds 40 minutes. On the basis of animal experimentation and clinical observation, DHCA, without additional neuroprotective measures is typically limited to no more than 60 minutes at 18°C (see Figure 10.1). Frustratingly, while some patients appear to tolerate DHCA >60 minutes without apparent injury, others sustain major brain injury after <20 minutes DHCA.

## Re-warming

Re-warming should be instituted following a planned rate of rise of core temperature. Excessively rapid re-warming, accompanied by a rise in cerebral arterio-venous $O_2$ difference, is known to worsen neurological outcome. In patients undergoing coronary artery bypass surgery, maintaining a temperature gradient of <2°C between inflow temperature and brain (nasopharyngeal) temperature has been shown to improve cognitive outcome. Because hyperthermia is known to exacerbate neuronal injury, inflow temperature should not exceed 37°C and CPB terminated when core body temperature reaches 35.5–36.5°C. A significant "afterdrop" is inevitable and patients are commonly admitted to the critical care unit with temperatures as low as 32°C. Using a slow rate of re-warming with adequate time for even distribution of heat between core and peripheral tissues helps to reduce the extent of this after-drop.

During the period of re-warming attention should be given to the correction of metabolic abnormalities, particularly the metabolic acidosis that inevitably accompanies reperfusion following circulatory arrest. Correction of acid–base balance may require the titrated administration of sodium bicarbonate or use of hemofiltration (ultrafiltration).

## Hemostasis

Prolonged CPB and hypothermia produce coagulopathy. Hemostasis is facilitated by meticulous surgery, the use of predonated autologous blood and administration of donor blood components under the guidance of laboratory tests of coagulation and thromboelastography. Despite safety concerns, antifibrinolytic agents (e.g., tranexamic acid, ε aminocaproic acid) and aprotinin have been shown to be efficacious in aortic arch surgery with DHCA. Recently published and widely publicized studies reporting a high incidence of adverse effects associated with aprotinin use in *adult* patients undergoing coronary revascularization and high-risk cardiac surgery have prompted withdrawal of the drug.

## Neuroprotection during DHCA

Although hypothermia is the principal neuroprotectant during DHCA, additional strategies may be employed to reduce the likelihood of neurological injury. These include: acid–base management strategy, hemodilution, leukodepletion and glycemic control. Surgical maneuvers, such as intermittent cerebral perfusion, selective antegrade cerebral perfusion (SACP) and retrograde cerebral perfusion (RCP), may also be used to both protect the brain and extend the operating time available to the surgeon (see Table 10.3).

## Hypothermia

Cerebral metabolism decreases by 6–7% for every 1°C fall in temperature below 37°C, with consciousness and autoregulation being lost at 30°C and 25°C, respectively. At temperatures <20°C, ischemic tolerance is around 10 times that at normothermia (see Figure 10.2). While some authors maintain that the EEG becomes isoelectric at this temperature, it is evident that a significant number of patients have measurable EEG activity at <18°C. In addition to its effects on metabolic rate, hypothermia appears to reduce lipid peroxidation, neuronal calcium entry, membrane depolarization, production of superoxide anions and the release of excitotoxic amino acids.

In many centers, ice packs or an ice-cold water jacket placed around the head after induction of anesthesia are used to augment cerebral cooling. The extent to which extracranial

**Table 10.3.** Neuroprotectant strategies during DHCA

| Anesthesia | Glycemic control |
| --- | --- |
| | External cranial cooling |
| | Neurological monitoring |
| | Cerebrospinal fluid drainage |
| | Pharmacological neuroprotection |
| Perfusion | Acid–base management strategy |
| | Hemodilution |
| | Leukocyte depletion |
| Surgical | Intermittent cerebral perfusion |
| | Selective antegrade cerebral perfusion (SACP) |
| | Retrograde cerebral perfusion (RCP) |

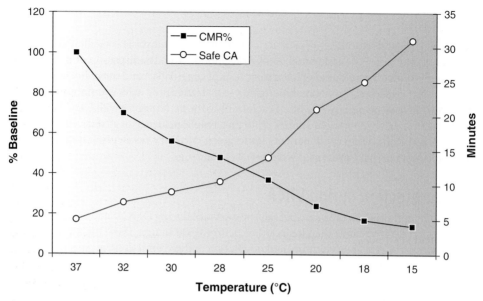

**Figure 10.2** The effect of temperature on cerebral metabolic rate (CMR%) and duration of safe circulatory arrest (CA). Data derived from McCullough *et al. Ann Thorac Surg* 1999; 67(6): 1895–9 and Kern *et al. Ann Thorac Surg* 1993; 56(6): 1366–72.

cooling influences brain temperature and neurological outcome in adult humans remains undocumented. Use of the procedure is justified on the basis of an absence of significant adverse effects and limited animal experimentation.

## Hemodilution

The combination of vasoconstriction, increased plasma viscosity and reduced erythrocyte plasticity secondary to hypothermia leads to impairment of the microcirculation and ischemia. Progressive hemodilution during hypothermic CPB, typically to a hematocrit of 0.18–0.20, is thought to partially alleviate this phenomenon. In some centers, a degree of normovolemic hemodilution is undertaken prior to the onset of CPB. The optimal hematocrit for a particular individual at a specific temperature remains unclear. Gross anemia (i.e., hematocrit <0.10) may result in inadequate oxygen delivery to tissues, particularly during re-warming. This approach is supported by the more recent observation that maintaining a higher hematocrit during deep hypothermic CPB did not impair the cerebral microcirculation.

## Acid–base management

Hypothermia increases the solubility of gases (e.g., $N_2$, $O_2$ and $CO_2$) in blood. While the total content of any particular gas in a blood sample remains constant, hypothermia shifts the equilibrium between dissolved and undissolved gas leading to an increase in the former, which in turn reduces the partial pressure of the gas. When analyzed at 37°C, a "normal" blood sample taken during hypothermia reveals "normal" results, whereas correction of these results for body temperature reveals reduced $PO_2$ and $PCO_2$, and alkalosis. Maintaining $PCO_2$ within the normal range on the basis of analysis at 37°C is termed *alpha-stat* management, whereas maintaining a normal $PCO_2$ (and pH) on the basis of "temperature-corrected" analysis is termed *pH-stat* management. This is discussed further in Chapter 6.

When cerebral perfusion pressure (CPP), $P_aO_2$ and $PCO_2$ are maintained within the physiological range, autoregulation couples cerebral blood flow (CBF) to cerebral metabolic rate ($CMRO_2$). Cerebral autoregulation is obtunded by profound hypothermia and hypercarbia. At $P_aCO_2 > 10$ kPa the classical autoregulation "plateau" is abolished and CBF becomes "pressure-passive" – dictated solely by CPP. Alpha-stat management preserves cerebral autoregulation and thus CBF decreases during hypothermia. By contrast, pH-stat management results in cerebral hyperperfusion, which in turn increases $O_2$ delivery and ensures more rapid and homogeneous brain cooling – albeit at the potential expense of increased microembolic load.

In the piglet model of DHCA, pH-stat management improves neurological outcome. In neonates undergoing DHCA for repair of congenital heart defects, pH-stat management prior to circulatory arrest appears to be associated with fewer complications than alpha-stat management and better developmental outcome. In adults, however, the superiority of one strategy over another in the setting of DHCA remains unproven. Alpha-stat management is used in many adult centers – presumably on the basis of superior cognitive outcome following hypothermic CPB, although some centers use a pH-stat strategy during cooling and an alpha-stat strategy during re-warming.

## Retrograde cerebral perfusion (RCP)

Reversing the direction of blood flow in the superior vena cava (SVC) has been advocated as a means of improving brain protection during DHCA and extending the period of "safe" DHCA. Following the onset of CPB, the cavae are snared and arterial blood directed into the SVC via an arterio-venous shunt constructed in the CPB circuit. Pump flows of 150–700 ml/minute are advocated to maintain a mean perfusion pressure of ~25 mmHg. The putative advantages of RCP include continuous cerebral cooling, cerebral substrate delivery and expulsion of air, particulates and toxic metabolites. The absence of blood flow detectable by transcranial Doppler in the middle cerebral arteries of a small, but significant number of patients subjected to RCP may explain conflicting evidence of efficacy. In addition, significant extracranial shunting via the external jugular veins may occur during RCP. Interestingly, the use of multi-modal neurological monitoring to guide RCP delivery at pressures as high as 40 mmHg – considered by many surgeons to be harmful – has shown this to be safe.

## Selective antegrade cerebral perfusion (SACP)

Selective hypothermic brain perfusion permits surgery to be conducted at lesser degrees of systemic hypothermia (e.g., 22–25°C). SACP often requires greater mobilization of the epiaortic vessels and division of the innominate vein. Following the onset of circulatory arrest, the aortic arch is opened and balloon-tipped arterial cannulae advanced into the innominate and left carotid artery ostia (see Figure 10.3). The left subclavian artery is clamped and arterial flow commenced at 10–20 ml/kg to maintain a perfusion pressure – measured in the right radial artery – of 50–70 mmHg. Alternative approaches include cannulation of the right subclavian artery and hemicerebral perfusion via the innominate artery alone. The technique provides more "physiological" cerebral perfusion, but has the disadvantage of increasing operative time and carries the risk of atheroembolism and microembolism. In a recently pub-

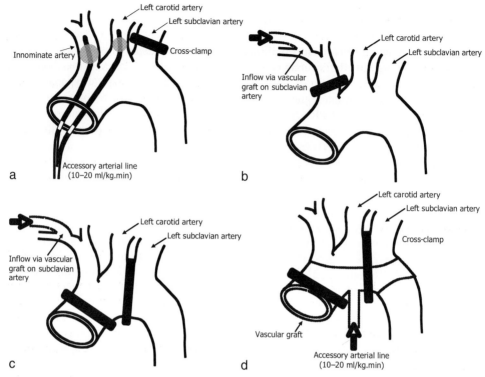

**Figure 10.3** Examples of selective antegrade cerebral perfusion techniques. (a) Direct cannulation of the innominate and left carotid arteries. (b) Hemicranial perfusion via a left subclavian artery graft. (c) Bilateral cranial perfusion via a left subclavian artery graft. (d) Bilateral cranial perfusion via a sidearm on vascular graft.

lished series of 501 consecutive patients undergoing aortic arch surgery with DHCA (25°C) and SACP (14°C), Khaladj *et al.* reported an overall mortality of 11.6% and permanent neurological deficit rate of 9.6%.

In some instances, intermittent, rather than continuous, antegrade cerebral perfusion is considered more practicable or expeditious. In a piglet model of DHCA, 1 minute of reperfusion for every 15 minutes of DHCA has been found to be sufficient to provide normal metabolic and microscopic cerebral recovery.

## Leukocyte depletion

The use of leukocyte-depleting arterial line filters is reported to moderate the systemic inflammatory response to CPB, reduce reperfusion injury and reduce postoperative infective complications. Evidence for cerebral protection by leukocyte depletion is lacking in humans and animal experimentation has yielded conflicting results.

## Glycemic control

Insulin resistance and hyperglycemia are common consequences of cardiac surgery and hypothermia. In animal models, hyperglycemia worsens cerebral infarction. Whilst tight glycemic control during cardiac surgery appears to reduce mortality and infective complications, any neuroprotective effect remains unproven.

## Spinal cord protection

Surgery involving the descending thoracic aorta may interrupt blood flow to the spinal cord via the anterior spinal artery (of Adamkiewicz) and cause paraplegia. Although drainage of cerebrospinal fluid (CSF) has long been proposed as a means of improving spinal cord perfusion, debate continues as to its efficacy. One early study suggested that postoperative hypotension – rather than avoidance of CSF drainage – was the only predictor of paraplegia. More recently, however, CSF drainage has been shown to reduce the incidence of paraplegia or paraparesis by 80% in a randomized study of 145 patients undergoing thoracoabdominal aortic aneurysm repair.

An alternative approach to spinal cord protection is the continuous infusion of ice-cold saline into the epidural space. Despite reports of efficacy, the technique has not been widely adopted.

## Pharmacological neuroprotection

At present no drug is specifically licensed for neuroprotection during cardiac surgery. Over the last four decades a wide variety of compounds, many with very promising preclinical pharmacological profiles, have been evaluated in the setting of cardiac surgery. These include anesthetic agents (barbiturates, propofol, volatile agents), calcium channel blockers, immunomodulators (corticosteroids, ciclosporin), amino acid receptor antagonists (magnesium, remacemide), glutamate-release inhibitors (lignocaine, phenytoin), antiproteases (aprotinin, nafamostat) and free radical scavengers (mannitol, desferrioxamine, allopurinol).

In many centers thiopental 15–30 mg/kg continues to be administered before DHCA despite any objective evidence of efficacy. The widely held belief that thiopental reduces neurological injury in conventional cardiac surgery is not borne out by the evidence, although there is some suggestion that it reduces overall mortality. Animal evidence suggests that the administration of corticosteroids (e.g., methylprednisolone 15 mg/kg) prior to DHCA affords a degree of neuroprotection. The recent demonstration of neuroprotection by sodium valproate in a canine model of DHCA has prompted a randomized trial of valproate in humans.

## Neurological monitoring

Until recently, the use of monitors of cerebral substrate delivery or neurological function (see Table 10.4) has largely been confined to specialist centers, researchers and enthusiasts. It goes without saying that a monitor must prompt a corrective intervention *before* the onset of irreversible neurological injury to be of any use. Cost and lack of level 1A evidence of efficacy means neurological monitoring has yet to be universally adopted as "standard of care."

### Substrate delivery

Fiberoptic jugular venous oxygen saturation ($S_jO_2$) monitoring provides a continuous measure of the global balance between cerebral oxygen supply and demand. The normal range for $S_jO_2$ is quoted to be 55–75%, but may be as high as 85% in some normal individuals. $S_jO_2 < 50\%$ is regarded as being indicative of inadequate cerebral oxygenation. A normal or near-normal $S_jO_2$ value may, however, mask regional cerebral ischemia; thus $S_jO_2$ monitoring has high specificity but low sensitivity for the detection of cerebral ischemia. $S_jO_2$ monitoring has been

**Table 10.4.** Neurological monitoring

| | |
|---|---|
| Clinical | Arterial pressure |
| | Central venous pressure |
| | CPB pump flow rate |
| | Arterial oxygen saturation |
| | Temperature |
| | Hemoglobin concentration |
| | Pupil size |
| | Arterial $PCO_2$ |
| Substrate delivery | Transcranial Doppler sonography |
| | Near infrared spectroscopy |
| | Jugular venous oxygen saturation |
| Cerebral activity | Electroencephalography |
| | Somatosensory evoked potentials |
| | Auditory evoked potentials |
| | Motor evoked potentials |
| Other | Epiaortic ultrasound |
| | Transesophageal echocardiography |

used to assess the adequacy of cerebral cooling prior to DHCA. Low $S_jO_2$ prior to the onset of DHCA is associated with adverse neurological outcome. $S_jO_2$ monitoring may also be used to monitor the adequacy of SACP.

In contrast to measuring cerebral $S_aO_2$ and $S_jO_2$, which provide a measure of global cerebral oxygen delivery and consumption, cerebral near infrared spectroscopy (NIRS) allows measurement of a region of tissue containing arteries, capillaries and (predominantly) veins (see Figure 10.4). Despite a lack of evidence of efficacy in adult cardiac surgery, NIRS is widely used in DHCA to assess cerebral oxygenation during cooling, DHCA and re-warming. Under deep hypothermic temperatures it is unclear what "normal" values for $S_jO_2$ and NIRS would be.

Transcranial Doppler (TCD) sonography has been mainly used as a surrogate measure of CBF and a means for detecting microemboli. In the setting of DHCA it has been used to monitor the adequacy of SACP, and assess autoregulation and CBF after surgery.

## Neurological function

Qualitative and quantitative EEG has been used in cardiac surgery for over 5 decades and has long been considered the "gold standard" for the detection of cerebral ischemia. Unfortunately, a consistent and reproducible EEG descriptor of reversible cerebral injury has remained frustratingly elusive. Although a sensitive indicator of neuronal injury, its use is complicated by the fact that hypothermia and virtually every anesthetic drug have profound influences on neuroelectrophysiology. Below 28°C there is progressive slowing until the EEG becomes isoelectric – a phenomenon used to assess the adequacy of cooling prior to DHCA. The temperature at which EEG activity is lost is subject to considerable inter-patient variation and is typically *higher* during the cooling phase than during re-warming.

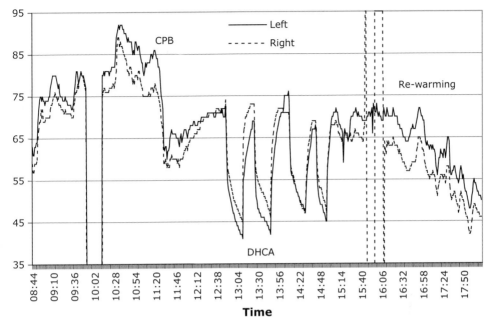

**Figure 10.4** Near infrared spectroscopy monitoring during pulmonary thromboendarterectomy. Significant cerebral desaturation is seen at the onset of CPB, during four periods of hypothermic circulatory arrest (DHCA), and during re-warming.

Evoked potential monitoring encompasses a number of techniques that measure the response of the nervous system to external stimulation. Sensory evoked potential monitoring techniques measure the cortical or brainstem responses to auditory, visual, spinal cord or somatic stimulation. Motor evoked potential (MEP) monitoring techniques measure the spinal cord or compound muscle action potential response to cortical stimulation. Abolition of specific components of the somatosensory evoked potential (SSEP) and brainstem auditory evoked potential (BAEP) have been used as a measure of cooling prior to DHCA.

## Postoperative care

Postoperative care is similar to that for any patient undergoing cardiac surgery. Every effort should be made to ameliorate the impact of secondary brain injury – hyperthermia, hypoxemia, hypotension and hypoperfusion should be aggressively treated. Even mild degrees of hyperthermia, a common occurrence after cardiac surgery, have been shown to be detrimental after DHCA.

## Outcome

The risks associated with DHCA are largely determined by the pathology being treated, the presence of significant comorbidities and the urgency of surgery.

Surgery with DHCA carries a finite risk of neurological injury. The type and pattern of neurological injury seen in neonates after DHCA appears to differ from that seen in older children and adults. In neonates, the predominant lesion is neuronal apoptosis in the hippocampus and the gray matter of the cerebral cortex. Seizures and choreoathetosis are by far the

137

most common clinical manifestations of neurological injury. By contrast, selective neuronal necrosis and infarction (i.e., stroke) in the cerebellum, striatum and neocortex are the predominant lesions in non-neonates. In a study of 656 patients undergoing DHCA, Svensson *et al.* reported an overall stroke rate of 7%. Univariate predictors of stroke included advanced age, a history of cerebrovascular disease, DHCA duration, CPB duration and concurrent descending thoracic aortic repair. In a study of 200 patients operated upon using DHCA between 1985 and 1992, Ergin *et al.* reported an in-hospital mortality of 15% and stroke rate of 11%. Age >60 years, emergency surgery, new neurological symptoms at presentation and permanent postoperative neurological deficits were found to be significant predictors of operative mortality. Stroke was more common in older patients and when the aorta was found to contain thrombus or atheroma. In 2008, a series of 347 DHCA patients from the Mayo Clinic was reported (Sundt *et al.* 2008). That investigation detailed DHCA as well as introduction of the protective adjuncts of retrograde or antegrade cerebral perfusion. For all patients mortality was 9% and stroke was 8%. Following that report the preferred approach at the Mayo Clinic is selective antegrade perfusion via the axillary artery, rather than retrograde cerebral perfusion.

## Suggested Further Reading

- Bigelow WG, Lindsay WK, Greenwood WF. Hypothermia; its possible role in cardiac surgery: an investigation of factors governing survival in dogs at low body temperatures. *Ann Surg* 1950; **132**(5): 549–66.

- Coselli JS, Lemaire SA, Koksoy C, Schmittling ZC, Curling PE. Cerebrospinal fluid drainage reduces paraplegia after thoracoabdominal aortic aneurysm repair: results of a randomized clinical trial. *J Vasc Surg* 2002; **35**(4): 631–9.

- Doblar DD. Intraoperative transcranial ultrasonic monitoring for cardiac and vascular surgery. *Semin Cardiothorac Vasc Anesth* 2004; **8**(2): 127–45.

- Dorotta I, Kimball-Jones P, Applegate R, 2nd. Deep hypothermia and circulatory arrest in adults. *Semin Cardiothorac Vasc Anesth* 2007; **11**(1): 66–76.

- Duebener LF, Sakamoto T, Hatsuoka S, *et al.* Effects of hematocrit on cerebral microcirculation and tissue oxygenation during deep hypothermic bypass. *Circulation* 2001; **104**(12 Suppl. 1): I260–4.

- Ergin MA, Galla JD, Lansman L, Quintana C, Bodian C, Griepp RB. Hypothermic circulatory arrest in operations on the thoracic aorta: determinants of operative mortality and neurologic outcome. *J Thorac Cardiovasc Surg* 1994; **107**(3): 788–97.

- Furnary AP, Wu Y, Bookin SO. Effect of hyperglycemia and continuous intravenous insulin infusions on outcomes of cardiac surgical procedures: the Portland Diabetic Project. *Endocr Pract* 2004; **10** (Suppl. 2): 21–33.

- Griepp RB, Stinson EB, Hollingsworth JF, Buehler D. Prosthetic replacement of the aortic arch. *J Thorac Cardiovasc Surg* 1975; **70**(6): 1051–63.

- Hoffman GM. Neurologic monitoring on cardiopulmonary bypass: what are we obligated to do? *Ann Thorac Surg* 2006; **81**(6): S2373–80.

- Hogue CW Jr, Palin CA, Arrowsmith JE. Cardiopulmonary bypass management and neurologic outcomes: an evidence-based appraisal of current practices. *Anesth Analg* 2006; **103**(1): 21–37.

- Khaladj N, Shrestha M, Meck S, *et al.* Hypothermic circulatory arrest with selective antegrade cerebral perfusion in ascending aortic and aortic arch surgery: a risk factor analysis for adverse outcome in 501 patients. *J Thorac Cardiovasc Surg* 2008; **135**(4): 908–14.

- Leyvi G, Bello R, Wasnick JD, Plestis K. Assessment of cerebral oxygen balance during deep hypothermic circulatory arrest by continuous jugular bulb venous saturation and near-infrared spectroscopy. *J Cardiothorac Vasc Anesth* 2006; **20**(6): 826–33.

- Priestley MA, Golden JA, O'Hara IB, McCann J, Kurth CD. Comparison of neurologic outcome after deep hypothermic circulatory arrest with alpha-stat and pH-stat cardiopulmonary bypass in newborn pigs. *J Thorac Cardiovasc Surg* 2001; **121**(2): 336–43.

- Rosomoff HL. The effects of hypothermia on the physiology of the nervous system. *Surgery* 1956; **40**(1): 328–36.

- Stecker MM, Cheung AT, Pochettino A, *et al.* Deep hypothermic circulatory arrest: I. Effects of cooling on electroencephalogram and evoked potentials. *Ann Thorac Surg* 2001; **71**(1): 14–21.

- Stier GR, Verde EW. The postoperative care of adult patients exposed to deep hypothermic circulatory arrest. *Semin Cardiothorac Vasc Anesth* 2007; **11**(1): 77–85.

- Sundt TM 3rd, Orszulak TA, Cook DJ, Schaff HV. Improving results of open arch replacement. *Ann Thorac Surg* 2008; **86**(3): 787–96.

- Svensson LG, Crawford ES, Hess KR, *et al.* Deep hypothermia with circulatory arrest. Determinants of stroke and early mortality in 656 patients. *J Thorac Cardiovasc Surg* 1993; **106**(1): 19–28.

# Organ damage during cardiopulmonary bypass

Andrew Snell and Barbora Parizkova

Cardiac surgery may be associated with deterioration in the function of a number of organ systems, commencing during surgery and persisting to varying degrees into the postoperative period. Organ damage during cardiac surgery has been primarily attributed to the use of cardiopulmonary bypass (CPB). Until recently it has been difficult to correctly distinguish the causative factors that are truly associated with CPB from those that result from surgery. Although CPB continues to be the most widely used technique for the conduct of cardiac surgical cases, there has been a resurgence of interest in the performance of coronary artery bypass grafting without CPB, termed "off-pump CABG" or OPCAB for short. The re-emergence of this technique has led to a number of studies evaluating organ function after cardiac surgery with and without the use of CPB and has resulted in an improvement in the quality of the available information regarding the role of CPB in causing organ dysfunction.

## Triggers of organ damage

The key mechanisms in causing organ damage associated with CPB are:

- the activation of a systemic inflammatory response (SIRS), which is an inevitable consequence of CPB;
- hemodilution and reduced blood viscosity, mainly at the onset of CPB, resulting in alterations in the distribution of blood flow to organs and flow characteristics of blood through capillary networks;
- ischemia/reperfusion injury to heart, lungs and organs supplied by the splanchnic circulation;
- laminar rather than pulsatile flow, although the significance of this remains controversial.

The cause, nature and severity of organ dysfunction in the context of cardiac surgery and CPB are described below in relation to each of the major organ systems. As cerebral and renal dysfunction are perceived to be the most frequent and debilitating consequences of CPB, they will be considered in separate chapters.

## SIRS

The principal causative mechanisms of SIRS associated with cardiac surgery are:

- activation of complement;
- activation of fibrinolytic and kallikrein cascades;
- synthesis of cytokines;
- oxygen radical production; and
- activation of neutrophils with degranulation and release of protease enzymes.

*Cardiopulmonary Bypass*, ed. S. Ghosh, F. Falter and D. J. Cook. Published by Cambridge University Press.
© Cambridge University Press 2009.

Transition from physiological circulation to CPB results in contact between blood and a number of non-biological surfaces that form the extracorporeal circuit. This, together with hypothermia, tissue trauma, organ ischemia and reperfusion and laminar flow, results in a very complex response involving the activation of complement, platelets, macrophages, neutrophils and monocytes. This massive, acute reaction initiates coagulation as well as the fibrinolytic and kallikrein pathways. The resulting SIRS is amplified by the subsequent release of endotoxins, cytokines, such as interleukins (IL) and tumor necrosis factor (TNF). Endothelial cell permeability is increased. Release of proteases and elastases is triggered by the subsequent migration of activated leukocytes into tissue. The parenchymal damage caused by this migration can exacerbate the ischemia/reperfusion injury associated with cardiac surgery (Figure 11.1)

The evident features of SIRS are coagulopathy, vasodilatation, and varying degrees of fluid shifts between the intravascular and the interstitial space, as well as the generation of

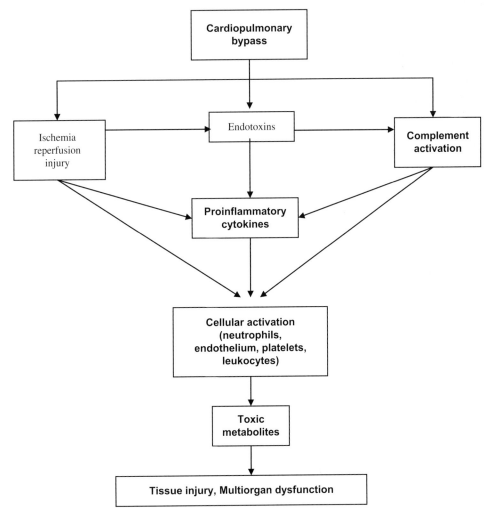

**Figure 11.1** Overview of the inflammatory response to CPB.

microemboli. The clinical effect is mostly a temporary dysfunction, to varying degrees, of nearly every organ system. However, SIRS can also be associated with major post-operative morbidity such as neurological, pulmonary, cardiac or renal dysfunction. It still remains unclear why two patients with similar physiological and perioperative variables may experience radically different degrees of this inflammatory response.

## Contact activation

Contact between blood and the components of the CPB circuit, in particular the oxygenator with its high surface area of synthetic material, and the direct exposure of blood to blood–gas interfaces, for example, gaseous bubbles, results in the activation of three inter-related plasma protease pathways:

- the complement pathway;
- the kinin–kallikrein pathway; and
- the fibrinolytic pathway.

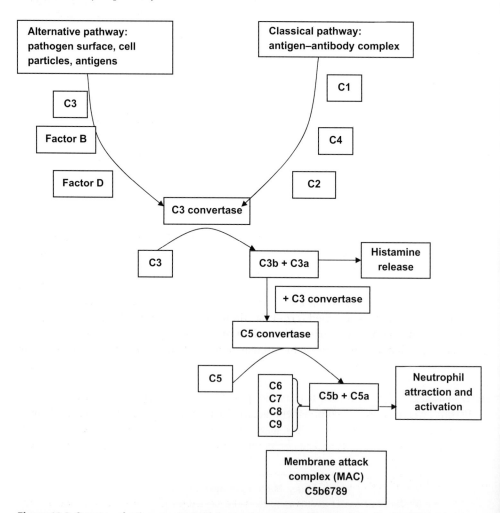

**Figure 11.2** Overview of pathways activated following the exposure of patients' blood to the CPB circuit.

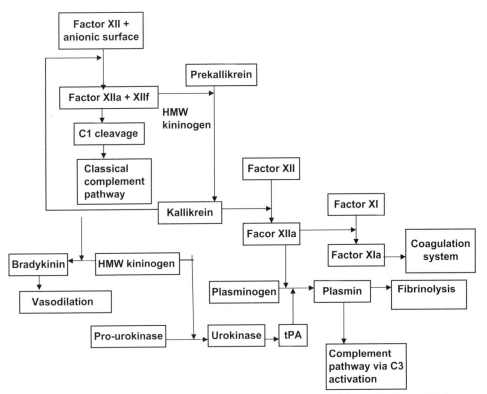

**Figure 11.3** Alternative and classical complement pathways are both activated during CPB. C3a and C5a, known as anaphylaxotoxins, stimulate mast cell degranulation and act as a chemoattractant for neutrophils.

## The complement system

The complement system consists of over 30 plasma proteins. Activation of complement causes cellular injury either by the direct actions of activated complement components or as a result of the activation of inflammatory cells by complement factors.

Activation of the system can occur through exposure to antigens, endotoxins or foreign surfaces, through either a "classical" or "alternative" pathway (see Figure 11.2). Cleavage of C3, by either route, to its activated form C3a stimulates the release of histamine and other inflammatory mediators from mast cells, eosinophils and basophils. This results in smooth muscle constriction and an increase in vascular permeability. C5a is a potent chemotactic factor for neutrophils; C5a promotes the aggregation, adhesion and activation of neutrophils. C3b and C5b interact on cell membranes with components C6–C9 to form a "membrane attack complex," which activates platelets and "punches" holes in cell membranes.

Plasma levels of activated complement factors rise within 2 minutes of the onset of bypass and a second rise can be detected after release of the aortic cross-clamp and on re-warming. Levels decline postoperatively and generally return to normal 18–48 hours postoperatively.

## The kinin–kallikrein pathway

Contact with anionic surfaces results in the activation of factor XII to its activated forms, factors XIIa and XIIf. In combination with high-molecular-weight kininogen (HMWK), factor

XIIa converts prekallikrein to kallikrein and, through a positive feedback loop, generates more factor XIIa. Kallikrein cleaves HMWK bound to surfaces to yield bradykinin. Bradykinin is a potent vasoactive substance that increases vascular permeability and promotes smooth muscle contraction and secretion of tissue plasminogen activator (see below). Kallikrein and factor XIIa cause neutrophil activation (see Figure 11.3).

## The fibrinolytic pathway

Fibrin clots formed at an incision site are eventually broken down by plasmin. Bradykinin promotes the production of tissue plasminogen activator (tPA), which converts plasminogen to plasmin. Plasma activity of tPA increases to its maximum within 30 minutes of CPB and usually returns to preoperative levels within 24 hours. In addition, kallikrein, in combination with HMWK, cleaves pro-urokinase to urokinase. Urokinase activates urokinase plasminogen activator (uPA), which causes more plasmin production. Plasmin proteolytically digests fibrin to form fibrin degradation products (FDPs). Fibrin degradation products further inhibit fibrin production and cause endothelial as well as platelet dysfunction.

Overall, thrombin formation and coagulation coincide with tPA release, plasmin formation and fibrinolysis. The effect is a state of global activation of thrombin formation, platelet consumption paired with the activation of fibrinolytic pathways.

## The role of the endothelium

Physiologically, endothelium plays a protective role by:

- secreting endogenous anticoagulants like tPA, thrombomodulin and heparin-like substances; and
- producing relaxing factors like NO and prostacyclin.

Endothelial cells can become injured in the presence of circulating cytokines, endotoxins, cholesterol, nicotine and sheer stress. Many cardiac patients will, therefore, have an activated endothelium prior to surgery.

CPB causes further activation through the triggered release of inflammatory cytokines, namely C5a, IL-1 and TNF. This will cause further expression of procoagulant and fibrinolytic enzymes as well as expression of membrane adhesion molecules, which will allow the transmigration of neutrophils and monocytes.

## Ischemia–reperfusion injury (IRI)

IRI is the term used to describe the cellular injury that occurs on resumption of normal perfusion to an organ after a period of relative or complete ischemia. During the ischemic period intracellular calcium accumulates due to the failure of ATP-dependent cellular pumps. On reperfusion, intracellular calcium levels further increase secondary to oxidative dysfunction of sarcolemma membranes. This cellular and mitochondrial calcium overload ultimately induces cardiomyocyte death by hypercontracture and opening of the mitochondrial permeability transition pores (PTP) on the inner mitochondrial membrane. Opening of the mitochondrial PTP channels during early reperfusion (they remain closed during the ischemic period) inhibits the mitochondrial membrane potential, uncoupling oxidative phosphorylation, which being essential for ATP production, results in ATP depletion and cell death. Large quantities of oxygen free radicals are generated on reperfusion of ischemic tissue. The oxygen free radicals, if present in sufficient concentration, overwhelm endogenous scavenging mechanisms and cause further intracellular injury. Oxygen free radicals also exacerbate arachidonic acid metabolism and the production of leukotrienes and thromboxanes, promoting aggregation, transmigration and activation of neutrophils to further compound the injury (see Figure 11.4). Neutrophils are the key final mediators of IRI by the production of toxic chemicals generated during the metabolism of oxygen and by the secretion of proteolytic enzymes released from granules stored in their cytoplasm.

During ischemia energy generation using high-energy phosphates (ATP) creates the metabolite hypoxanthine, which has a tendency to accumulate. The enzyme *xanthine dehydrogenase* normally metabolizes hypoxanthine. Under conditions of ischemia followed by rapid reperfusuion, *xanthine dehydrogenase* is converted to *xanthine oxidase* as a result of the higher availability of oxygen. This oxidation results in molecular oxygen being converted into highly reactive superoxide and hydroxyl radicals. Excessive nitric oxide produced during reperfusion reacts with superoxide to produce the potent free radical peroxynitrite. These radicals attack cell membrane lipids, proteins and DNA, causing further damage.

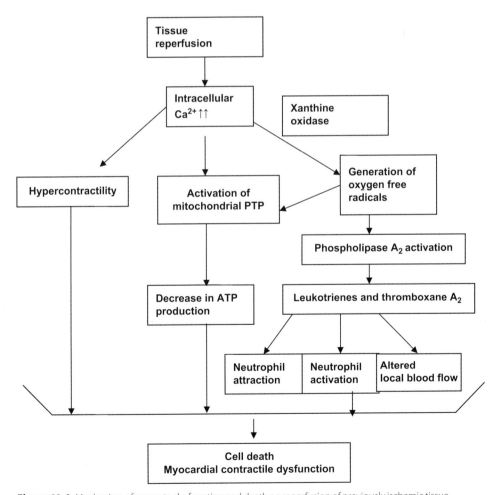

**Figure 11.4** Mechanism of myocyte dysfunction and death on reperfusion of previously ischemic tissue.

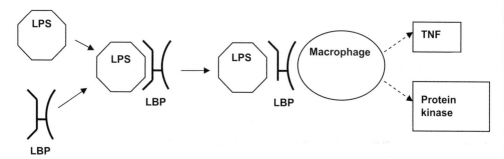

**Figure 11.5** The role of endotoxins from gut translocation in the pathogenesis of the inflammatory response to CPB. Lipopolysaccharides (LPS) bind to LPS-binding protein (LBP). This complex activates macrophages releasing TNF and protein kinase.

## Endotoxins

The plasma levels of endotoxins increase during CPB. Endotoxins are lipopolysaccharides (LPS) derived from the cell membranes of gram-negative bacteria. The source of the endotoxins is widely believed to primarily be the gastrointestinal tract. Reduction in blood flow through the splanchnic circulation during CPB and the SIRS associated with CPB and aortic cross-clamping may result in a breakdown of the mucosal barrier in the gastrointestinal tract with consequent translocation of endogenous bacteria into the circulation.

The subsequent breakdown of bacterial cells releases LPS, which are bound to LPS-binding protein (LBP). The LPS–LBP macromolecular complex is a highly potent activator of macrophages, which release TNF and protein kinase, thus exacerbating SIRS further (see Figure 11.5).

## Therapeutic strategies

A number of strategies have been employed to ameliorate the extent of the SIRS seen during CPB.

- Pharmacological: using steroids prior to the onset of CPB, antioxidants and proteolytic enzyme inhibitors. None of these interventions have had clinically meaningful impact.
- Heparin-bonded circuitry can be used with the intention of reducing the degree of complement activation, but has proven to be less effective in attenuating coagulation or fibrinolysis.
- Hemofiltration/ultrafiltration (convection and osmosis under hydrostatic pressure) has been incorporated into the circuitry to remove low-molecular-weight substances from plasma with the aim of reducing the circulating levels of proinflammatory mediators. Current techniques have proven to be more effective in the pediatric than the adult population.
- Leukocyte-depleting filters incorporated in the CPB circuit, to reduce the number of circulating activated white cells. Their value is presently unclear, but leukocyte depletion may have a protective effect in reducing the severity of lung and myocardial injury observed post-CPB. The most consistent benefit is found in higher risk patients with pre-existing lung disease, ventricular dysfunction or those receiving long CPB times.

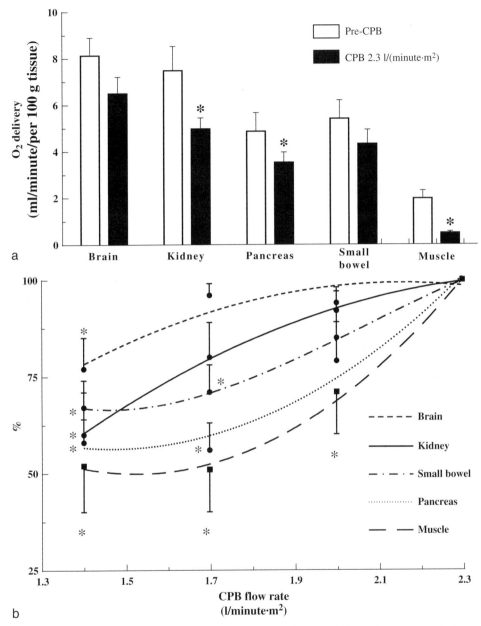

**Figure 11.6** (a) Regional $O_2$ delivery with onset of cardiopulmonary bypass. (b) Change in organ $DO_2$ with changes in flow rate (Q). Mean values ± SE *$p$ <0.05 versus CPB at 2.3 l/minute/$m^2$.

- Leukocytes in allogenic blood transfusions have important immunomodulatory effects in the recipient. The use of leukocyte depleted stored blood has been shown to decrease mortality in some patients who undergo CPB. This is predominantly due to a decrease in non-cardiac causes of death, in particular multiorgan failure.

## CPB versus OPCAB

Off-pump CABG is an alternative technique for coronary revascularization, which is still controversial and highly dependent on institutional preference. Clinical reports have shown that oxidative stress and markers of inflammation (particularly IL-8, TNF and E-selectin) are significantly reduced during OPCAB when compared to CABG performed on CPB. OPCAB has also been shown to be associated with a reduction in blood transfusion. Full heparinization may be avoided during OPCAB and this, together with the avoidance of hemodilution by the priming volume required for CPB, may be more important in reducing transfusion requirements than any advantageous effects from ameliorating SIRS.

## Alterations in organ perfusion

The distribution of blood flow to organs is altered on transition from physiological circulation to CPB and thus oxygen delivery also alters (see Figure 11.6a). Furthermore, tissue oxygen delivery is influenced to a large extent by CPB flow rate (see figure 11.6b). Organ dysfunction may, thus, be in part attributed to these changes in the regional distribution of blood flow and the dependence of oxygen delivery on the maintenance of adequate CPB flow rates.

## Gastrointestinal complications

Gastrointestinal (GI) complications are reported as occurring in 2–4% of patients following cardiac surgery. There is a high associated mortality rate of about 30%; GI complications account for about 15% of all cardiac surgical deaths.

GI complications usually present as GI bleeding, peritonitis or acute bowel obstruction with abdominal distension. Perforation or ischemic bowel is a common finding. Often, the earliest presenting sign is a progressive metabolic acidosis. Bleeding from the upper GI tract accounts for almost 30% of all GI complications after cardiac surgery and is far more common than bleeding from the lower GI tract. Lower GI tract bleeding is usually associated with bowel ischemia or pre-existing large bowel disease.

CPB causes profound reductions in blood flow in the splanchnic circulation and thus leads to reduced perfusion to the GI tract and associated organs. Gastrointestinal mucosal blood flow is reduced and remains reduced for several hours postoperatively. This may be further exacerbated by the use of vasoconstrictors during CPB and by embolization of atheromatous debris from the aorta or clot from the heart into the mesenteric circulation. Severe intestinal ischemia may occur during CPB even when the indices of global body perfusion remain normal. The release of a variety of vasoactive factors during CPB, such as vasopressin, catecholamines and thromboxanes, lead to a redistribution of regional blood flow away from the mucosa of the GI tract.

The combination of reduced splanchnic blood flow and the CPB-induced SIRS reduce the efficacy of both the absorptive and barrier functions of the GI tract. The increase in gastrointestinal mucosal permeability results in the translocation of bacterial endotoxins from the GI tract into the bloodstream, amplifying SIRS and subsequent further organ damage. Risk factors associated with adverse gastrointestinal (GI) outcome are summarized in Table 11.1.

## Hepatic dysfunction

Hepatic metabolism is reduced during CPB in conjunction with the reduction in splanchnic blood flow. Hepatic blood flow has been reported to decrease by 19% after CPB is commenced.

**Table 11.1.** Risk factors associated with adverse gastrointestinal (GI) outcome

| Variable | Models for adverse GI outcome ($n = 133$): odds ratio (95% CI) | | |
| --- | --- | --- | --- |
| | Preoperative model | Intraoperative model | Both models |
| Increased preoperative total bilirubin >1.2 mg/dl* | 2.4 (1.2–4.9) | | 2.5 (1.2–5.0) |
| Combined cardiac procedures | 2.9 (1.8–4.5) | | 2.0 (1.3–3.2) |
| Preoperative platelets 130 000/μl | 2.9 (1.3–6.4) | | 2.8 (1.3–6.2) |
| Previous cardiovascular surgery | 3.0 (1.9–4.7) | | 2.2 (1.4–3.4) |
| Preoperative EF <0.4* | 1.9 (1.2–3.0) | | 1.7 (1.1–2.6) |
| Age >75 years | 1.8 (1.1–2.9) | | |
| Preoperative PTT >37 seconds | 2.0 (1.3–3.1) | | 1.7 (1.1–2.5) |
| Pharmacological cardiovascular support | | 1.9 (1.3–2.9) | 2.0 (1.3–3.2) |
| Intraoperative transfusion of PRBCs | | 1.9 (1.6–2.3) | 1.7 (1.4–2.1) |
| Intraoperative circulatory failure | | 1.7 (1.1–2.6) | |
| Aortic cross-clamp time | | 1.5 (1.0–2.3) | |

CI = confidence interval; EF = ejection fraction; PTT = partial thromboplastin time; PRBCs = packed red blood cells.
* Missing data were included as low risk on justification.
Adapted from Multicenter Study of Perioperative Ischemia Research Group. Anesth Analg 2004; 98: 1610–17.

There may be a transient rise in the levels of hepatic enzymes measured in the blood, which usually peaks early in the postoperative period. Clinically evident jaundice is only apparent in a small number of patients, although bilirubin levels rise in about 20% of cases. Moderate or severe degrees of hepatic dysfunction are rare and usually occur in concert with multiorgan failure.

There is poor correlation between preoperative hepatic function and the risk of developing postoperative hepatic dysfunction. Consequences of hepatic dysfunction relevant to CPB specifically include:

- impaired drug metabolism;
- reduced plasma protein concentrations leading to reduced plasma oncotic pressure and alteration in the volume of distribution of drugs;
- impaired coagulation due to reduction in production of clotting factors; and
- impaired ability to generate heat and regulate temperature.

Cholecystitis, in the absence of gall stones, may also occur postoperatively in 0.2–0.5% of all cardiac surgical patients. The gall bladder distends and the stasis of bile leads to inflammation of the gall bladder; it carries a mortality rate of 25–45% once diagnosed, despite aggressive treatment.

# Pancreatitis

Overt pancreatitis, characterized by a rise in serum amylase to over 1000 IU/l, occurs in 0.1–1% of cases following cardiac surgery. Lesser degrees of pancreatic cellular injury with mild elevations in serum amylase concentrations are, however, common. The etiology is probably related to perioperative reduction in splanchnic blood flow causing pancreatic ischemia. Risk factors for developing postcardiac surgical pancreatitis are:

- prolonged CPB;
- perioperative hypotension;
- low postoperative cardiac output;
- hypothermia; and
- perioperative administration of large quantities of $Ca^{2+}$.

$Ca^{2+}$ administration, frequently used to treat intraoperative hypertension, has not clearly been identified as an independent risk factor.

Uncomplicated pancreatitis carries a mortality of 5–10%, but cases that progress to necrotizing pancreatitis or to the development of abscesses or a pseudocyst usually result in death.

There is limited evidence that OPCAB surgery has significant benefits over cardiac surgery with CPB in preventing GI complications

## Pulmonary dysfunction

Cardiac surgery results in impairment of gas exchange for a variety of reasons. While most patients will display subclinical functional changes, the incidence of post-CPB acute respiratory disease syndrome (ARDS) is <2%. The mortality rate associated with post-CPB ARDS, however, is >50%. The principal causes of postoperative respiratory failure are:

- atelectasis;
- increase in lung water content as a result of:
  - increased capillary permeability caused by SIRS
  - impaired hemodynamics in the immediate postoperative period
  - the additional fluid load during CPB;
- alterations in the production of surfactant, particularly during the period of lung collapse during CPB and as a result of SIRS;
- transfusion-related acute lung injury (TRALI);
- altered chest wall mechanics resulting from sternotomy;
- decreased static and dynamic lung compliance;
- pneumothorax or hemothorax; and
- phrenic nerve injury impairing diaphragmatic function.

Although some of the factors listed above relate to cardiac surgery in general and are not specific to CPB, the overall effect is the development of intrapulmonary shunts that cause a mismatch between ventilation and perfusion. This manifests as a higher inspired oxygen concentration being required to maintain an acceptable level of blood oxygenation. This mismatch tends to resolve gradually postoperatively, but patients may require supportive measures such as the application of PEEP during mechanical ventilation or continuous positive airway pressure (CPAP) when spontaneously breathing until resolution occurs. The maintenance of adequate tidal volumes without reaching excessive airway pressures during supported respiration may help to limit atelectasis. The administration of diuretics as an adjunct to careful fluid balance may help to reduce interstitial lung water.

Lung injury may be more evident following cardiac surgery in patients with pre-existing lung disease and in smokers.

The therapeutic interventions investigated have had little or no effect on postoperative lung function:

- steroid administration before CPB fails to prevent poor postoperative lung compliance;
- leukocyte depleting filters in the CPB circuitry show inconsistent effects on post-CPB lung function;
- heparin-coated circuits and continuous hemofiltration on CPB improve pulmonary vascular resistance and transpulmonary shunting in a transient and clinically insignificant way; and
- maintaining mechanical ventilation on CPB does not lead to any significant preservation of lung function.

There is conflicting evidence as to the benefits of avoiding CPB and electing for OPCAB in terms of postoperative pulmonary dysfunction. However, there is a suggestion that patients with chronic pulmonary disease benefit from OPCAB more in terms of preservation of lung function than those with no significant pre-existing lung disease.

## Myocardial dysfunction

The period of CPB during cardiac surgery can be divided into three phases:

- onset of CPB until application of the cross-clamp;
- the period of cross-clamping and cardioplegic or fibrillatory arrest; and
- the reperfusion period following removal of the cross-clamp and ultimately separation from CPB.

During these periods the heart is subjected to injury from microemboli, the inflammatory products of SIRS, regional hypoperfusion, complete ischemia and finally reperfusion injury. The injurious effects incurred from these insults, together with the potential for inadequate myocardial protection and distension of the flaccid heart during the period of cross-clamping, result in myocardial edema and reduced ventricular contractility, which may continue into the postoperative period. Furthermore, if the heart is subject to excessive preloading or high afterloading during weaning from CPB, left ventricular end-diastolic volume, myocardial wall stress and oxygen consumption are all increased, further contributing to deterioration in cardiac function.

OPCAB avoids the need for cross-clamping of the aorta and for cardioplegia, which are both essential during CABG with CPB. In theory, this should minimize the risk of global myocardial ischemia and myocardial stunning. In practice, the incidence of myocardial infarction is similar following OPCAB and CABG with CPB. OPCAB, however, is associated with a more rapid recovery of myocardial oxidative metabolism and this leads to more rapid replenishment of myocardial high-energy phosphates such as ATP and so to better myocardial function in the early postrevascularization phase.

## Quality of life

The ultimate measure of the success of a medical intervention is its ability to improve the quality of life for patients. There is much evidence to show that both mental and physical health are improved after cardiac surgery and furthermore studies comparing quality of life after cardiac surgery with CPB or OPCAB yield similar results. This is a testament to the fact that CPB provides a safe and effective means for performing cardiac operations.

## Suggested Further Reading

- Laffey JG, Boylan JF, Cheng DCH. The systemic inflammatory response to cardiac surgery. *Anesthesiology* 2002; **97**: 215–52.

- McSweeney ME, Garwood S, Levin J, *et al.* Adverse gastrointestinal complications after cardiopulmonary bypass: can outcome be predicted from perioperative risk factors? *Anesth Analg* 2004; **98**: 1610–61.

- Ng CSH, Wan S, Yim APC, *et al.* Pulmonary dysfunction after cardiac surgery. *Chest* 2002; **121**: 1269–77.

- Ngaage DL. Off-pump coronary artery bypass grafting: the myth, the logic and the science. *Eur J Cardiothor Surg* 2003; **23**(4): 557–70.

- Sellke FW, DiMaio M, Caplan LR, *et al.* Comparing on-pump and off-pump coronary artery bypass grafting. *Circulation* 2005; **111**: 2858–64.

- Wan S, LeClerc J, Vincent J. Inflammatory response to cardiopulmonary bypass: mechanisms involved and possible therapeutic strategies. *Chest* 1997; **112**: 676–92.

- Yellon DM, Hausenloy DJ. Myocardial reperfusion injury. *N Engl J Med* 2007; **357**:1121–35.

**Chapter**

**12**

# Cerebral morbidity in adult cardiac surgery

David Cook

## Neurological complications in adult cardiac surgery

Postoperative brain injury has been a focus of attention since the inception of cardiac surgery. In the last decade, approximately 2000 English-language articles have been published in this area. However, there has been only a modest decrease in the incidence of stroke or encephalopathy and the syndrome of cognitive dysfunction may be more prevalent today than 20 years ago. In fact, McKhann, comparing stroke incidence in 1994 (2.9%) and in 2004 at Johns Hopkins Hospital in Baltimore found a greater incidence in 2004 (4.5%) presumably because of the greater level of pre-existing disease in the more recent group of patients presenting for cardiac surgery. A great deal, however, has been learned about brain physiology and mechanisms of injury in cardiac surgery; changes in practice have occurred that are probably making neurological outcomes better than might be predicted, given the increasing age and associated medical conditions prevalent in the surgical population.

In the 1980s and 1990s, a large number of physiological and clinical studies were conducted that better characterized brain physiology and function during cardiac surgery and cardiopulmonary bypass (CPB). The physiological variables that were investigated as possible causes of perioperative brain injury included mean arterial pressure (MAP), body temperature, hematocrit (HCT), bypass pump flow rate, the use of pulsatile flow and $CO_2$ management. During this same period pharmacological and physiological interventions and changes in surgical technique were also investigated with an eye to reducing neurological morbidity. While many of those investigations can be faulted for being statistically underpowered, two decades of research have not led to either a brain protectant drug or device that has become part of our routine practice and substantially improved neurological outcomes. In fact, there is little evidence that intraoperative physiological management itself is an independent determinant of neurological outcome.

## Cerebral physiology during cardiopulmonary bypass

The results of a large number of investigations can be best summarized by saying that in adults, over the range of conditions in which nearly all CPB is conducted, the determinants of cerebral blood flow and metabolism are the same as those under non-bypass conditions.

CPB may profoundly affect cerebral blood flow (CBF) and cerebral metabolic rate of oxygen consumption ($CMRO_2$), but these changes are qualitatively no different from those that would occur under non-CPB conditions; they are simply quantitatively greater. During CPB conducted above 27°C, which constitutes about 90% of adult surgery, brain physiology is straightforward and predictable. However, when bypass is conducted under moderately to profoundly hypothermic conditions some of these relationships change, primarily because of the non-linearity of changes in $CMRO_2$ and a relative cold-induced vasoparesis.

*Cardiopulmonary Bypass,* ed. S. Ghosh, F. Falter and D. J. Cook. Published by Cambridge University Press.
© Cambridge University Press 2009.

The determinants of cerebral perfusion during cardiopulmonary bypass are, in order of importance:

- mean arterial blood pressure;
- hematocrit;
- cerebral metabolism; and
- $P_aCO_2$.

The absence of pulsatility does not determine CBF nor does pump flow, independent of its effect on MAP.

In the past there was considerable confusion over the effect of mean arterial pressure on cerebral perfusion during CPB. This arose from the poor design of studies conducted in the 1980s and a failure to appreciate the profound effect that changes in HCT have on cerebral blood flow. At least two very prominent studies from the 1980s concluded that CBF was independent of MAP, to MAPs as low as 30–40 mmHg during CPB. This conclusion was based on pooling very few measurements of CBF from large numbers of patients. Because the measurements were conducted at multiple MAP, temperature, HCT and $PCO_2$ conditions, in multiple patients, a great deal of scatter was demonstrated in the data. When regression analysis relating MAP and CBF was performed on the widely scattered data, no relationship between MAP and CBF could be identified. The study design was thus not adequate to test the hypothesis and the conclusion was misleading.

The other primary source of confusion about the relationship between MAP and CBF arose from a failure to appreciate the profound effect of HCT on CBF. A variety of investigations determined CBF before CPB. Then during CPB, at a significantly lower MAP (below 55 mmHg), CBF measurements were repeated and found to be nearly the same as CBF at a higher MAP prior to CPB. These studies failed to take into account the fact that significant hemodilution occurs during CPB and that this reduces blood viscosity and increases CBF. This was well elucidated by Plöchl and Cook who randomized exposure to varying MAP in dogs during CPB at 33°C and found that, while CBF was increased for any given degree of hemodilution, CBF and cerebral oxygen delivery decreased when MAP fell below approximately 55 mmHg (see Figure 12.1).

After MAP and HCT, cerebral metabolism is a primary determinant of cerebral blood flow. Over the temperature range where most adult bypass is conducted, 27°C to 37°C, there is a clear relationship between temperature, $CMRO_2$ and CBF. Below 25°C, the relationships become much more complex. If all other variables (primarily MAP, HCT and $CO_2$) are controlled, a 10°C decrease in temperature reduces $CMRO_2$ by about 50% and this is associated with a 50% reduction in CBF.

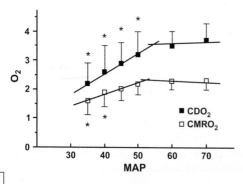

**Figure 12.1** Cerebral oxygen delivery ($CDO_2$) and cerebral oxygen consumption ($CMRO_2$) versus mean arterial pressure (MAP) during cardiopulmonary bypass (CPB) at 33°C. Values for oxygen (on ordinate in ml/100 g per minute) are the mean ± standard deviation (*P <0.05 versus MAP of 60 mmHg by repeated-measure analysis of variance followed by Student–Neuman–Keuls test). (From Plöchl W, Cook DJ, Orszulak TA, et al. Critical cerebral perfusion pressure during tepid heart surgery in dogs. Ann Thorac Surg 1998; 66: 118–124, with permission.)

$P_aCO_2$ is an independent determinant of CBF during bypass. However, during most adult cardiac surgery the effect of $P_aCO_2$ is relatively small. If all other variables are controlled, every 1 torr increase or decrease in $P_aCO_2$ alters CBF approximately 3%. As such, between 32°C and 37°C the maximal effect of $CO_2$ on CBF is about 15%. The effect of $CO_2$ and alpha-stat/pH-stat strategies becomes increasingly relevant below 27°C, but it is a minor consideration above 32°C.

Cerebral physiology during CPB has been somewhat difficult to determine because so many variables are subject to change simultaneously and some of the physiological variables interact. This is clear in the interactions of HCT, MAP and CBF. The same physiological linkage of variables also leads to confusion about the effect of pump flow on CBF. Some literature has reported that cerebral perfusion is dependent on pump flow. This misunderstanding arose from the failure to appreciate that pump flow, like cardiac output, is a primary determinant of mean arterial pressure. While decreases or increases in CBF may be seen when pump flow is increased or decreased, this is really only clearly demonstrated below or near the autoregulatory threshold: above a MAP of approximately 55 mmHg, increases in pump flow do not increase CBF, while below about 55 mmHg reductions in pump flow result in reductions in MAP that then lead to reductions in CBF. This was well demonstrated in an animal study by Sadahiro (see Figure 12.2).

The dependence of CBF on pump flow is seen only when pump flow is too low to generate a MAP above the autoregulatory threshold. In humans and in animals, the independence of

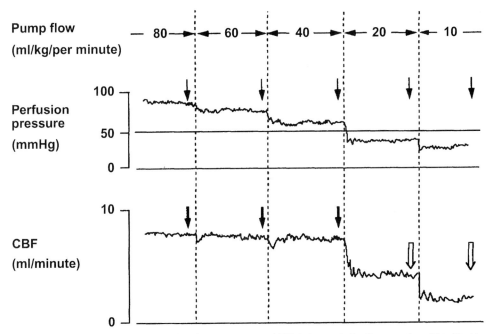

**Figure 12.2** Continuous monitoring of perfusion pressure and CBF during perfusion flow rates from 80 to 10 ml/kg/minute. Arrows indicate the point at which the relationship between CBF and perfusion pressure was evaluated. Black arrows show the presence of an autoregulatory response with CBF returning to its prior level after an initial drop. White arrows show the loss of a vascular response. (From Sadahiro M, Haneda K, Mohri H. Experimental study of cerebral autoregulation during cardiopulmonary bypass with or without pulsatile perfusion. *J Thorac Cardiovasc Surg* 1994; 108: 446–454, with permission.)

**Table 12.1.** Effect of pump flow on cerebral perfusion

| 30 adult patients, CPB at 27°C | High flow | Low flow |
|---|---|---|
| Pump flow (l/minute/m²) | 2.3 ± 0.1 | 1.2 ± 0.1 |
| MAP (mmHg) | 63 ± 9 | 62 ± 6 |
| CBF (ml/100g/minute) | 29 ± 7 | 30 ± 8 |

From Cook DJ, *et al. Cardiothorac Anesth* 1997; 11: 415–9 with permission.

CBF from pump flow between 1.2 and 2.3 l/minute/m²) at a stable MAP has been well shown at 27°C (see Table 12.1).

Pulsatile flow appears to have no effect on cerebral blood flow during CPB independent of any effect of pulsatility on MAP.

# Intraoperative ischemia and physiological management

For strokes initiated in the operating room, watershed infarcts constitute the minority of cerebral ischemic events. When available, neuroimaging usually demonstrates embolic events and associated regional hypoperfusion. This is probably why, in spite of intensive clinical and laboratory study, it has been difficult to show that physiological variables, such as temperature or perfusion pressure, during CPB are independent determinants of neurological outcome. For intraoperative strokes it is more likely that these variables modulate the severity of injury that occurs subsequent to a cerebral embolic event. Because of the frequency of cerebral ischemic events, physiological management remains a relevant part of practice even if it does not prevent most strokes.

## Effect of perfusion pressure

Through much of the 1980s the surgical, and some of the anesthesia literature, indicated that the cerebral autoregulatory threshold was shifted leftward during bypass such that lower mean arterial pressures (35–40 mmHg) were capable of maintaining normal cerebral blood flow. This was incorrect. Although hemodilution associated with CPB increases cerebral blood flow for any given mean arterial pressure, the autoregulatory curve still "breaks" at a pressure of approximately 55 mmHg; below this level cerebral blood flow is compromised. A combination of well-conducted laboratory investigations, the clinical investigation by Gold and colleagues showing better composite cardiac and neurological outcomes at higher mean arterial pressures, and a better understanding of cerebral autoregulation in the elderly, patients with diabetes and hypertensives have led clinical practice to maintain MAPs above 55–60 mmHg during CPB. Rather than preventing watershed infarcts, this practice helps to maintain cerebral perfusion in the presence of carotid, cerebral and penetrating vessel disease and supports collateral flow and perfusion of the peri-ischemic region when embolic events do occur.

## Effect of temperature on neurological outcome

Given the profound effects of temperature on cerebral oxygen demand and the widely held belief in the neuroprotective effect of hypothermia, it was reasonable to expect that absolute CPB temperature would be identified as a primary determinant of cognitive outcome. However, this has not been the case in randomized or non-randomized trials. Although there are "multiple" publications investigating the effect of perioperative temperature management on neurological outcomes, the weight of the evidence is far weaker than would be expected. This is not to say that perioperative temperature management is unimportant, only that the best evidence of an effect of a hypothermic management on neurological outcome is quite weak. Whilst the debate over the relative benefits of hypothermic versus normothermic bypass remain unresolved, more detailed examination of the influence of re-warming rate and post-operative temperature in determining cognitive outcomes have produced interesting results.

Data from the 2001 Grigore study randomizing intraoperative temperature management was reported again when a subset of that negative outcome trial was used to examine the effect of re-warming speed on cognitive outcomes. The cognitive data was analyzed as a continuous variable (better or worse) as well as a dichotomous variable (defect present or not). Univariate analysis did not show a re-warming effect on cognitive outcome, nor did treatment of cognitive outcome as a dichotomous variable in multivariate analysis. However, the authors concluded that slow re-warming had a positive effect because analysis of cognitive outcome data as a continuous variable was associated with greater improvement in cognitive performance than conventional re-warming.

The simplest improvement in clinical practice relating to temperature management during CPB followed the first documentation of cerebral hyperthermia in 1996. Cook et al. showed that brain temperature was systematically underestimated during CPB and that cerebral temperature can approach 40°C during re-warming, a period associated with a great number of embolic events. From this observation, closer monitoring of nasopharyngeal and perfusate temperature and prevention of hyperthermia during CPB have become a standard part of intraoperative care.

## Effect of glucose control

Maintaining blood glucose in the normal range is more a matter of not doing harm than actually doing something to prevent or reverse ischemic injury. The experimental stroke literature clearly demonstrates that hyperglycemia, like hyperthermia, worsens neurological outcome in the event of an ischemic insult. So while maintaining perioperative normoglycemia will not independently determine the incidence of perioperative stroke, it is very likely to moderate its severity when ischemia does occur.

## Effect of other measures

Few other intraoperative interventions hypothesized to improve neurological outcome have found their way into clinical practice. A range of different classes of drugs have been tried including aprotinin, complement inhibitors, steroids, barbiturates, propofol, xenon, calcium channel antagonists and magnesium, to name but a few. None has proved efficacious in a sufficiently powered clinical trial.

## Perioperative stroke

Stroke is one of the most devastating complications following adult cardiac surgery. Literature from the 1960s and 1970s indicates that the incidence of stroke was around 2–4%. When one looks at very large populations, reports from the last 5 years demonstrate that this is largely unchanged. The overwhelming risk factor for stroke is physiological age, particularly manifest as atherosclerotic disease. In the 1990s a great deal of attention was paid to whether physiological variables were responsible for neurological outcomes, but none of these studies produced compelling evidence. With the rapid expansion of echocardiography and transcranial Doppler studies, attention shifted towards intraoperative embolization as the primary etiology of perioperative stroke and cognitive dysfunction.

While difficult to measure, due to lack of a concurrent control group, improvements in surgical technique have probably restricted the rise in incidence of stroke, which would have been anticipated in the ageing population of patients, with more complex medical conditions, presenting for cardiac surgery. Thus, even if overall stroke incidence in cardiac surgery is relatively unchanged, at least it has not risen to the levels that outcome models would predict. Recognition of the importance of embolic stroke has led to increased care in handling of the ascending aorta. Transcranial Doppler, echocardiographic and neuroimaging data all point to the ascending aorta as the primary cause of intraoperative stroke. Intraoperative imaging, single application of the aortic clamp, femoral cannulation, all-arterial grafting and off-pump techniques that eliminate ascending aorta instrumentation probably all reduce intraoperative embolization. However, even with excellent surgical management of the ascending aorta there still remains a substantial incidence of perioperative brain injury. This is best exemplified in off-pump CABG during which the aorta is not manipulated.

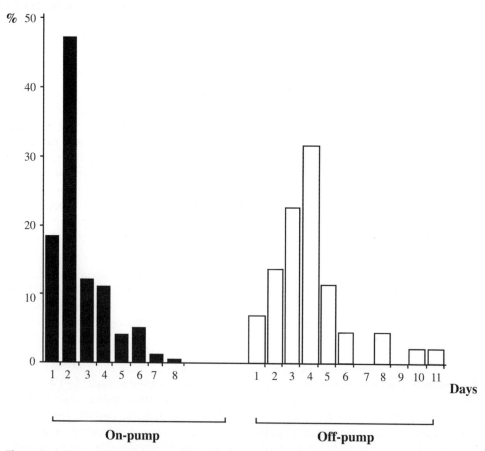

**Figure 12.3** Chronological distribution of the onset of postoperative stroke for on-pump and off-pump CABG. (From Garrett K, Peel MHS, Sotiris C, et al. Chronological distribution of stroke after minimally invasive versus conventional coronary artery bypass. J Am Coll Cardiol 2004; 43: 752–6, with permission.)

## Off-pump CABG (OPCAB) and stroke

Off-pump CABG evolved from minimally invasive surgery and a desire to eliminate any morbidity associated with CPB. There was an expectation that elimination of CPB would dramatically eliminate perioperative strokes. Interestingly, this has not been fully borne out. Stroke rates vary greatly in cardiac surgical reports depending on the patient population and the type of surgery; however, in single institution CABG surgery, aortic "no touch techniques" or off-pump surgery seem to only moderately reduce stroke risk. In a compelling study of over 16 000 patients, Bucerius described a stroke rate of 3.9% in CABG with conventional bypass versus 2.5% in the off-pump group. A similar effect of off-pump surgery is identified by Peel and colleagues who in a study population of almost 3300 off-pump and 7300 on-pump CABG found a stroke rate of 1.35% in off-pump and a 2.4% in on-pump CABG (see Figure 12.3). This effect of eliminating aortic instrumentation, about a 1% decrease in stroke incidence, is similar to what has been described in a large off-pump meta-analysis as well as the stroke reduction identified with surgical management guided by epiaortic scanning. This moderate but meaningful effect is important because it indicates that more than half of perioperative strokes may not be related to intraoperative embolization from the aorta. The limited neuroimaging data available support this: brain imaging shows a 30% incidence of subclinical cerebral ischemic events in OPCAB.

There are also data to suggest that strokes that occur with off-pump and on-pump CABG have different timing.

## Timing of cardiac surgery-related stroke

Given the low incidence of perioperative stroke, the vast majority of clinical studies have been retrospective to attain study populations of sufficient size. They typically identify a discharge code for stroke and have rarely identified the timing of an adverse cerebral event. However, one of the most important publications on perioperative stroke in cardiac surgery demonstrated that more than 50% of perioperative strokes occurred postoperatively (see Figure 12.4). This has been confirmed in at least three subsequent investigations from other institutions. In one retrospective study of 10 573 patients, nearly 73% of strokes occurred after the patient had woken from surgery without neurological deficit. The implications of this observation have not been fully appreciated and are important because the etiology and prevention of early and delayed stroke are likely to be different. As such, current bias towards intraoperative interventions would have an impact on less than 50% of the strokes observed in practice.

Using multivariate analysis in a study population of 1172, Zingone and colleagues found that early strokes were significantly more frequent in patients with ascending aortic atherosclerosis while delayed strokes were most strongly predicted by patient age. Reinforcing this was their observation that aortic scanning and changing surgical technique had far greater impact on early stroke than on delayed stroke. A conclusion of this study was that for the majority of late strokes a plausible mechanism, different from aortogenic embolism, could be identified. The most prominent of mechanisms were postoperative CPR and atrial fibrillation (AF). Comparison of stroke data in on-pump and off-pump CABG is also supportive of precipitating events. Peel and colleagues looked at stroke timing in on-pump and off-pump CABG patients and found that on-pump CABG was associated with earlier events than off-pump CABG.

The origin of delayed strokes may also be embolic, but relatively little research has gone into investigating their etiology or prevention. Apart from rarer interventions such as

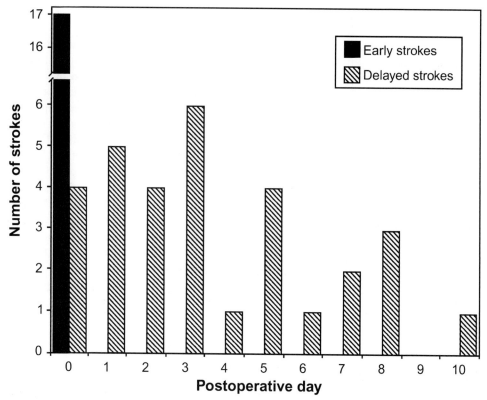

**Figure 12.4** Number of strokes detected immediately after surgery (early strokes) and after initial uneventful neurological recovery (delayed strokes) by day neurological event was detected. Note: postoperative day 0 refers to day of surgery, which begins after arrival in intensive care unit. (Hogue CW Jr, Murphy SF, Schechtman KB, Dávila-Román VG. Risk factors for early or delayed stroke after cardiac surgery. Circulation 1999; 100: 642–647, © 1999 American Heart Association, Inc.)

ventricular assist devices or cardiac arrest with CPR, postoperative stroke might result from aortic plaques, which become unstable at the time of surgery, or embolism of cardiac thrombi related to sludging in the left atrium due to AF or generalized left atrial enlargement.

In the geriatric general cardiology population, AF has a high incidence of associated stroke with clot formation in the left atrium, occurring early after the onset of AF. In cardiac surgical patients, the overall incidence of AF is about 25% and in some populations the incidence of new onset AF can be as high as 60%. Data from a variety of sources indicate that postoperative AF may be responsible for at least 30% of late strokes. In studies separating early and late strokes, multivariate analysis consistently shows that postoperative AF is an independent predictor of late stroke and has been reported to be associated with a six-fold increase in stroke risk. The mean time of postoperative occurrence has typically been identified as postoperative day 3 or 4. In addition to thromboembolic risk from an atrium in fibrillation, postoperative stroke may also result from thrombus formation associated with regional wall motion abnormalities or from thrombus originating on left heart suture lines. This is more likely in low cardiac output states. Prophylactic therapy with antiplatelet drugs, such as aspirin, postoperatively may thus improve neurological as well as cardiac outcomes in certain groups of cardiac surgical patients (see Figure 12.5).

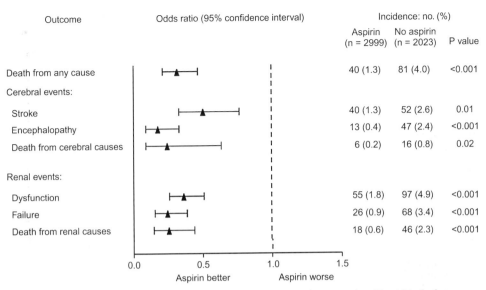

**Figure 12.5** Fatal and non-fatal ischemic outcomes amongst patients who received aspirin within the first 48 hours and patients who did not. The number of patients at risk varied with the type of outcome, since outcomes occurring within 48 hours after surgery were excluded from the analysis. A total of 73 patients had multiple causes of death. (Modified with permission from Mangano DT, *et al. N Engl J Med* 2002; 347: 1309–17, figure 1.)

# Stroke risk in the general population

History of a prior cerebral ischemic event is one of the most powerful predictors of perioperative stroke in cardiac surgery. In the study by Hogue and coworkers, prior stroke increases the risk of an early perioperative stroke by almost 12-fold and the risk of a delayed stroke by nearly 28-fold, which suggests that delayed stroke may be more related to patient-intrinsic risk factors than specific intraoperative events (see Table 12.2).

The general population has a background incidence of stroke risk factors, in particular:

- Hypertension;
- atrial fibrillation;
- diabetes; and
- prior stroke.

The practice of cardiology concentrates the highest risk general population patients under its care and often refers the worst of those to cardiac surgery. As such, the risk of stroke and renal disease is progressively distilled from general internal medicine to cardiology and then into the cardiac surgical population.

The American Heart Association provides population statistics for major cardiovascular disorders and the 2008 report identifies an overall stroke prevalence of 2.6% in the general population. The prevalence of stroke in 60–79 year-olds is about 6.3% and close to 13% in those aged over 80. Even more specific for understanding neurological injury in cardiac surgery is the incidence of annual hospital stroke admissions for diabetic and non-diabetic patients (see Figure 12.6), which shows that for diabetic patients over age 65 their annual likelihood of hospital admission for stroke is 3–7%. This population data places the incidence of perioperative stroke in an important light. It indicates that the likelihood of perioperative stroke (generally thought of as 2–4% in moderate-risk patients) is nearly identical to the

**Table 12.2.** Strokes classified depending on whether the neurological deficit was identified either immediately after surgery (early events) or after initial uneventful neurological recovery (delayed events)

| Variable | Odds ratio (95% CI) | P |
|---|---|---|
| Early strokes | | |
| History of stroke | 11.6 | <0.001 |
| Female sex | 6.9 | 0.004 |
| Ascending aorta atherosclerosis | 2.0 | 0.004 |
| Cardiopulmonary bypass time | 1.1 | 0.005 |
| Delayed strokes | | |
| History of stroke | 27.6 | <0.0001 |
| Diabetes | 2.8 | 0.008 |
| Female sex | 2.4 | 0.028 |
| Low cardiac output syndrome and atrial fibrillation | 1.7 | 0.033 |
| Ascending aorta atherosclerosis | 1.4 | 0.047 |

Odds ratio reflects risk of stroke with increase in a single level in the aortic scan results. The odds of an increase of 2 levels (e.g., normal to moderate/severe) is the square of the reported odds ratio.
From Hogue CW, *et al. Circulation* 1999; 100: 642–7, table 6 with permission.

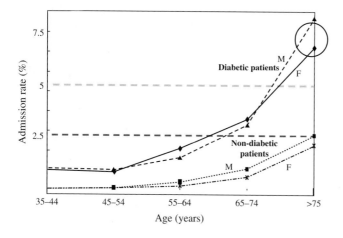

**Figure 12.6** Age- and sex-specific annual admission rates for cerebrovascular disease (CVD) in patients with and without diabetes in the general UK population. (Modified with permission from Currie CJ, Morgan, CL, Gill L, Stott NCH, Peters JR. *Stroke* 1997; 28: 1142–6, © 1997 American Heart Association, Inc., figure 1.)

annual risk in the general population. This is not to say that cardiac surgery isn't responsible for strokes; however, it is helpful to consider that the perioperative experience may be precipitating the existing stroke risk. If we think of cardiac surgery as precipitating pre-existing, population-based risk, very important parallels with neurological and renal dysfunction following cardiac surgery are evident.

In the general population, those who have had transient ischemic attacks (TIAs) have an approximately 50% chance of stroke within the next 6 months and an approximately 10% risk of another stroke within 2 years. In fact, the predictive value of prior stroke on all major adverse cardiovascular outcomes is profound, particularly in low-income patients (see Table 12.3). Table 12.3 shows the high incidence of recurrent stroke and mortality from

**Table 12.3.** Cumulative occurrence of secondary events in Medicare sample by cohort and type of secondary event

| Time since initially identified event, y | Stroke cohort (n = 1518) type of secondary event (%) | | |
|---|---|---|---|
| | AMI | Stroke | OVD |
| 0.5 | 0.7 | 3.7 | 0 |
| 1 | 1.6 | 6.2 | 0 |
| 2 | 3.4 | 10.8 | 0.3 |
| 3 | 5.1 | 12.2 | 1.8 |

AMI = acute myocardial infarction; OVD = other vascular death.
Modified with permission from Vickrey BG, et al. Stroke 2002; 33: 901–6, table 4.

cardiovascular causes in those who have had a prior stroke. These are the population-based risks independent of hospitalization, interventional cardiology or cardiac surgery.

While cardiac surgeons are reluctant to take patients to the operating room with recent stroke (primarily because of hemorrhagic risk), the clinical implications of a history of cerebrovascular events are underappreciated. A Cleveland Clinic study analyzed 126 patients with prior stroke undergoing cardiac surgery. They demonstrated that 17% of patients who had had a stroke within 3 months before surgery had a new perioperative stroke while those with prior stroke more than 3 months before surgery had a 12% incidence of new perioperative stroke. In patients with perioperative strokes, those with a more recent history of stroke appeared to be more sensitive to perioperative hypotension than those with more remote events, suggesting persistent cerebral vulnerability of these patients to hemodynamic instability.

Placing cardiac surgical stroke in the context of the stroke risk in the general population strongly suggests that:

- the most profound determinant of neurological outcome is the patient's previous medical history rather than specific intraoperative event; and
- a large proportion of adverse outcomes may result from the precipitation or triggering of patient risk factors by events in the perioperative period.

## Neurocognitive outcomes in cardiac surgery

If we think of perioperative stoke as being intimately related to pre-existing population-based risk, similar observations can be made for postoperative cognitive change. Postcardiac surgical cognitive decline has been an area of intense interest for the last 10 years. Depending on the assessment tools, study timing and design, the incidence of early postoperative cognitive change is 35–85% with longer term dysfunction seen in up to 10–30% of patients. It has also been suggested that the perioperative cardiac surgical experience was responsible for worsened cognitive status 5 years following surgery.

Because cognitive change is far more frequent than stroke it became the endpoint of many outcomes trials in the last several years. However, no intervention has resulted in a clinically meaningful reduction in its incidence. The most likely intervention to reduce cognitive injury should be off-pump surgery because exposure to CPB and instrumentation of the ascending aorta is eliminated. However, randomized studies with sufficient numbers of patients have failed to show a clinically meaningful effect. The trial by Van Dijk randomized patients to CABG on or off pump. At 3-month follow up, 21% of off-pump and 29% of on-pump patients

**Table 12.4.** Randomized 142 off-pump, 139 on-pump CABG cognitive assessment at 3 and 12 months

| Incidence of cognitive decline (%) | 3 months (P = 0.15) | 12 months (P = 0.69) |
|---|---|---|
| Off-pump | 21 | 30.8 |
| On-pump | 29 | 33.6 |

From Van Dijk D, *et al. JAMA* 2002; 287(11): 1405–12 with permission.

**Table 12.5.** Mean changes in z-scores for coronary artery bypass graft patients and PCI controls for the eight cognitive domains

| Domain | Baseline to 3 months: CABG vs. controls | 3 to 12 months: CABG vs. controls |
|---|---|---|
| Verbal memory | P >0.017 | ns |
| Visual memory | ns | ns |
| Language | ns | ns |
| Attention | ns | ns |
| Visuoconstruction | ns | ns |
| Psychomotor | ns | ns |
| Motor speed | ns | ns |
| Executive | ns | ns |

From Selnes OA, *et al. Ann Thorac Surg* 2003; 75(5): 1377–84 with permission.

showed cognitive decline, while at 1 year follow up decline had occurred in 31% of off-pump and 34% of on-pump patients (see Table 12.4).

Most studies have concluded that off-pump CABG has better cognitive outcomes, but the differences between groups appear to be so small as to be of limited clinical importance.

Several other observations place cognitive change following cardiac surgery in a perspective outside of perioperative injury. Firstly, there is an incidence of cognitive change after major non-cardiac surgery. While of a lower incidence, the character of the cognitive change is the same and in these other types of surgery there is no CPB and little or no risk of cerebral ischemia. Secondly, long-term cognitive outcomes in percutaneous coronary intervention (PCI) patients appear to be no different from those in patients undergoing CABG (see Table 12.5). This is important because CABG and PCI patients are very closely matched for patient (or population) risk factors of age, atherosclerosis, diabetes and hypertension. If cognitive outcomes at 1 year are the same in these PCI and CABG populations, it suggests that the longer term cognitive changes described following cardiac surgery are probably an expression of chronic brain changes related to those comorbidities rather than the cardiac surgery itself. Cook and colleagues used diffusion MRI and cognitive testing to document perioperative cerebral ischemia in cardiac surgical patients. They found that approximately 30% of patients showed ischemic changes indicative of postoperative cerebral embolization; however, there was no relationship between perioperative ischemic events and either in-hospital or postdischarge cognitive dysfunction (see Figure 12.7). The incidence of cognitive dysfunction was exactly the same whether or not patients had experienced a cerebral ischemic event. Furthermore, MRI data was suggestive that the cognitive decline was more a function of chronic

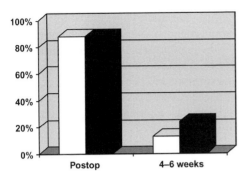

**Figure 12.7** Incidence of cognitive decline in cardiac surgery patients with and without acute cerebral ischemia ( □ = ischemia; ■ = no ischemia.), P <0.05. (From Cook DJ, *et al*. Post cardiac surgical cognitive impairment in the aged using diffusion-weighted magnetic resonance imaging. *Ann Thorac Surg* 2007; 83: 1389–95, figure 2, with permission.)

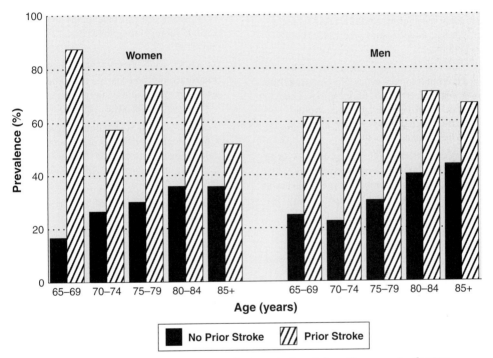

**Figure 12.8** Prevalence of MRI infarct by sex, age and prior stroke. Association with age was significant at $P < 0.0001$ in men and women without prior stroke; sex association was not significant in those without prevalent stroke ($P > 0.1$). Neither sex nor age associations were significant in those with prior stroke. (From Price TR, *et al. Stroke* 1997; 28: 1158–64, figure 1, with permission.)

ischemic microvascular disease than of a perioperative event. This would be consistent with growing neurology literature on chronic organic brain disease, cognition and occult cerebral ischemia in the general elderly population.

Two large studies have used neuroimaging to identify the incidence of occult cerebral ischemia in older cardiology patients: The Cardiovascular Health Survey conducted more than 3000 cerebral MRIs in community cardiology patients and the Rotterdam Scan Study carried out more than 1000 MRIs. These studies found that approximately 20–40% of the general population over age 60 have evidence of occult, small-vessel cerebral infarction (see Figure 12.8). This appears to be the result of penetrating vessel disease due to chronic hypertension, diabetes and atherosclerotic disease. Separate studies have linked this type of chronic small vessel ischemia to vascular dementia and cognitive change. As such, the cognitive changes seen following cardiac surgery may be the manifestation of underlying chronic brain disease unmasked in the perioperative period by drugs, metabolic changes, sleep deprivation and environmental changes rather than an expression of a perioperative insult. From this perspective it would also follow that cognitive declines seen 5 years after surgery are the evolution of underlying chronic brain disease rather than the evolution of an insult occurring in the perioperative period.

## Suggested Further Reading

- Chertow GM, Levy EM, Hammermeister KE, *et al.* Independent association between acute renal failure and mortality following cardiac surgery. *Am J Med* 1998; **104**(4): 343–8.

- Cook DJ. Neurologic effects of cardiopulmonary bypass. In Gravlee GP, ed. *Cardiopulmonary Bypass: Principles and Practice*, 3rd ed. Philadelphia: Wolters Kluwer Health/Lippincott Williams & Wilkins; 2008: 376–408.

- Cook DJ, Oliver WC, Jr, Orszulak TA, *et al.* Cardiopulmonary bypass temperature, hematocrit, and cerebral oxygen delivery in humans. *Ann Thorac Surg* 1995; **60**(6): 1671–7.

- Cook DJ, Orszulak TA, Daly RC, *et al.* Cerebral hyperthermia during cardiopulmonary bypass in adults. *J Thorac Cardiovasc Surg* 1996; **111**: 268–9.

- Cook DJ, Proper JA, Orszulak TA, *et al.* Effect of pump flow rate on cerebral blood flow during hypothermic cardiopulmonary bypass in adults. *J Cardiothor Vasc Anesth* 1997; **11**: 415–9.

- Gold JP, Charlson ME, Williams-Russo P, *et al.* Improvement of outcomes after coronary artery bypass. A randomized trial comparing intraoperative high versus low mean arterial pressure. *J Thorac Cardiovasc Surg* 1995; **110**: 1302–11.

- Hix JK, Thakar CV, Katz EM, *et al.* Effect of off-pump coronary artery bypass graft surgery on postoperative acute kidney injury and mortality. *Crit Care Med* 2006; **34**(12): 2979–83.

- McKhann GM, Grega MA, Borowicz LM Jr, *et al.* Stroke and encephalopathy after cardiac surgery: an update. *Stroke* 2006; **37**(2): 562–71.

- Mehta RL, Cantarovich F, Shaw A, *et al.* Pharmacologic approaches for volume excess in acute kidney injury (AKI). *Int J Artif Organs* 2008; **31**(2): 127–44.

- Peel GK, Stamou SC, Dullum MK, *et al.* Chronologic distribution of stroke after minimally invasive versus conventional coronary artery bypass. *J Am Coll Cardiol* 2004; **43**(5): 752–6.

- Plöchl W, Cook DJ. Quantification and distribution of cerebral emboli during cardiopulmonary bypass in the swine: the impact of $PaCO_2$. *Anesthesiology* 1999; **90**(1): 183–90.

- Plöchl W, Cook DJ, Orszulak TA, *et al.* Critical cerebral perfusion pressure during tepid heart surgery in dogs. *Ann Thorac Surg* 1998; **66**: 118–24.

- Sadahiro M, Haneda K, Mohri H. Experimental study of cerebral autoregulation during cardiopulmonary bypass with or without pulsatile perfusion. *J Thorac Cardiovasc Surg* 1994; **108**: 446–54.

- Shaw PJ, Bates D, Cartlidge NEF, *et al.* An analysis of factors predisposing to neurological injury in patients undergoing coronary bypass operations. *Q J Med* 1989; **72**: 633–46.

# Chapter 13

# Acute kidney injury (AKI)

Robert C. Albright

The incidence of perioperative renal injury appears to be increasing in the ever more complex elderly population presenting for cardiac surgery. More often than not acute kidney injury (AKI) is associated with well-defined risk factors that precede the surgical event. AKI complicates cardiovascular surgery in as many as 30% of all procedures, leading to dramatically worse outcomes, including increased mortality and substantial financial cost.

The incidence of AKI requiring dialysis among patients who undergo coronary artery bypass grafting alone is roughly 1%. However, when valve surgery or coronary artery bypass grafting and valve surgery occur concomitantly, the risks of AKI requiring dialysis are 1.7 and 3.3%, respectively. The risks for AKI rise substantially with the severity of chronic kidney disease (CKD), which afflicts as many as 30 million people in the USA.

## Definitions

Lack of a universally accepted definition of the syndrome of acute renal failure has hampered the study, understanding, management and prevention of this disastrous complication. The complexities of the accompanying fluid, electrolyte, acid–base and azotemic solute accumulation have led to approximately 50 different diagnostic criteria for acute renal failure to be cited in the literature.

A subgroup of intensivists and critical care nephrologists has formed the AKI Outcomes and Quality Study Group. This group has agreed upon a new definition of acute renal injury, which replaces "acute renal failure" and enhances the recent Risk, Injury, Failure, Loss, End stage ("RIFLE") criteria. Acute kidney injury has replaced the previous term of acute renal failure.

An abrupt decline in kidney function over less than 48 hours as defined by an increase in serum creatinine of 0.3 mg/dl (greater than 25 μmol/l) or a 50% increase over baseline accompanying a decreased urine output of less than 0.5 ml/kg/hour is generally accepted as a definition of AKI.

- **Stage I** – As an increase in serum creatinine of greater than 0.3 mg/dl or greater than 150% increase in baseline and urine output of 0.5 ml/kg/hour for 6 hours.
- **Stage II** – A serum creatinine increase of greater than 200–300% over baseline with concomitant decreased urine output to <0.5 ml/kg/hour for the past 12 hours.
- **Stage III** – An increase in serum creatinine greater than 300% over baseline, or an absolute level of greater than 4 mg/dl, accompanying a urine output of <0.3 ml/kg/hour) for the past 12 hours. Also included within the stage III definition would be any patient who requires renal replacement therapy.

*Cardiopulmanory Bypass*, ed. S. Ghosh, F. Fatter and D. J. Cook. Published by Cambridge University Press.
© Cambridge University Press 2009.

However, even this new definition is limited by the utilization of increasing creatinine as the serum marker of decreased renal function (decreased glomerular filtration rate, GFR). Increased serum creatinine is well known to lag significantly behind the development of acute injury, and is confounded by its dependence on tubular secretion and relationship to muscle mass and catabolism. Biomarkers of AKI, including serum and urine neutrophil gelatinase-associated lipocalin (NGAL), serum cystatin C, interleukin 17 (IL-17) and kidney injury marker-1 (KIM-1), are relatively new markers of kidney injury and poor kidney function. NGAL has been shown to be an excellent predictor of AKI in the pediatric population, specifically in the cardiovascular surgical population. Serum and urinary increases in NGAL preceded increase in creatinine by over 2 days. Importantly, among pediatric cardiovascular surgical patients with AKI, NGAL is very specific as well. Unfortunately, NGAL and the other currently studied newer biomarkers in general are not specific enough in the adult population to be of use as yet.

## Outcomes associated with AKI

It is difficult to overstate the negative clinical impact AKI portends when occurring in association with cardiovascular surgery. Any AKI occurring in the perioperative period carries an accompanying mortality rate of 15–30%, increasing substantially to at least 50% when dialysis is required. In fact, an adjusted covariant-independent observation of an eight-fold increase in death rate has been reported among a large cohort of cardiovascular surgical patients (see Table 13.1).

Even slight decreases in GFR imply an increased mortality risk. A 30% decrease in GFR found during the perioperative period is associated with a 6% overall morality over the subsequent year, as compared with 0.4% mortality without an accompanying AKI. A relative increased mortality risk of four- to five-fold with any increase in serum creatinine has additionally been reported among patients followed for 1 year.

When dialysis is required for AKI, recovery of renal function sufficient to discontinue chronic dialysis occurs in less than half of these patients. This obviously leads to a dramatic decrease in quality of life and longevity (20% mortality rate per year).

The cause of death associated with AKI is most often infection. In fact, approximately 58% of patients with AKI requiring perioperative dialysis in the cardiovascular surgery arena have a diagnosis of sepsis as compared to 3.3% of those without AKI. Whether the sepsis was the cause or result of the AKI is not determined in these studies.

The risks for bleeding, wound complications and nutritional compromise are also increased among patients with AKI.

**Table 13.1.** Influence of renal dysfunction and AKI on the incidence (%) of mortality and duration of intensive care unit and hospital stay (LOS) (in days) after coronary revascularization

|  | Mortality (%) | ICU LOS (days) | Hospital LOS (days) |
| --- | --- | --- | --- |
| Normal renal | 0.9 | 3.1 | 10.6 |
| Renal dysfunction | 19.0 | 6.5 | 18.2 |
| AKI | 63.0 | 14.9 | 28.8 |

Adapted from Mangano CM, Diamonstone LS, Ramsey JG, et al. Renal dysfunction after myocardial revascularization: risk factors, adverse outcomes and hospital utilization. *Ann Intern Med* 1998; 128: 194–203.

# Risk factors for AKI

Generally, the risk factors for developing AKI can be separated into those that are patient related versus those that are procedure related. Patient-related factors are predominant, once again emphasizing the overwhelming consequences of the ageing population with their concomitant increased burden of chronic illness. The most important patient-related issue predicting AKI is pre-existing chronic kidney disease. There is an overall 10–20% risk of AKI requiring dialysis among cardiac surgical patients with a serum creatinine preoperatively of 2–4 mg/dl, and the risk of requiring dialysis increases to nearly 28% with a preoperative serum creatinine of greater than 4 mg/dl.

The proportional impact of pre-existing subclinical renal insufficiency is extremely well illustrated by the decade-old study by Chertow. In a study of 43 000 patients, Chertow used multivariate analysis to identify independent risk factors for dialysis in cardiac surgical patients. A fraction of his data is presented in Table 13.2. Of greatest importance is the profound effect of moderately reduced creatinine clearance (CrCl) on the likelihood of postoperative dialysis. In this study of over 40 000 patients, approximately 60% had a CrCl less than 80 ml/minute. As such, 60% of the population has an odds ratio for dialysis that is equal to or greater than the increase in odds ratio seen with the risk factor of prior heart surgery. The weight of the numbers is astonishing. Anesthetists and surgeons think of prior heart surgery as a profound risk factor, but Chertow demonstrates that moderate decreases in preoperative CrCl is as potent a predictor of postoperative dialysis. Even more important, there are five times as many patients with subclinical renal insufficiency as those who undergo redo operations. Given the "normal" declines in CrCl seen as adults age from 65 to 80 years, the importance of this risk factor cannot be overestimated.

**Table 13.2.** Laboratory evaluation of acute kidney injury

|  | Prerenal | Intrinsic Renal | Postrenal |
|---|---|---|---|
| BUN/Cr ratio | >20 | 10–20 | 10–20 |
| Urine specific gravity | >1.020 | ~1.010 | >1.010 early, <1.0101 late |
| Uosmol (mosmol/kg) | >350 | ~300 | >400 early, ~300 late |
| U Na (mEq/l) | <20 | >30 | <20 early, >40 late |
| FE Na (%) | <1* | >2–3 | <1 early, >3 late |
| U Cr/P Cr ratio | ≥40 | ≤20 | >40 early, ≤20 late |
| Urine microscopy | Normal, hyaline casts | ATN: dark granular casts, hyaline casts, renal epithelial cells/casts | |
|  |  | GN: RBCs, dysmorphic RBCs (>20%), RBC casts, WBC/WBC casts, proteinuria | |
|  |  | AIN: urine eosinophilia, WBC, WBC casts, hyaline casts (consider CES) | |

AIN = acute interstitial nephritis; ATN = acute tubular necrosis; BUN = blood urea nitrogen; CES = cholesterol emboli syndrome; Cr = creatinine; FE Na = fractional excretion of sodium (calculated as: U Na/P Na × P Cr/U Cr × 100); GN = glomerulonephritis; P Cr = plasma creatinine; P Na = plasma sodium; U Cr = urinary creatinine; U Na = urinary sodium; Uosmol = urinary osmolality.
*Falsely low FE Na seen occasionally with acute GN, radiocontrast nephropathy, rhabdomyolysis.

Other associated risk factors from a patient perspective include pre-existing diabetes mellitus, female gender, increasing age, preoperative congestive heart failure, peripheral vascular disease, preoperative balloon pump requirements, chronic obstructive pulmonary disease, emergency surgery, anemia and, although somewhat controversial, decreased serum ferritin level.

Whether on-pump versus off-pump cardiac surgery may afford increased risk for AKI has been recently evaluated. Overall, a propensity matched trial has found that on-pump CABG carries a risk of AKI of approximately 2.6% versus 1.2% when surgery is performed off-pump. Difficulties in weaning from CPB and postoperative intra-aortic balloon pump (IABP) are intuitive additional risks for AKI.

No single etiological factor is responsible for the development of postoperative ARF, but a number of related factors probably interact to contribute to cause renal injury.

## Etiology of AKI

In this context, the principal etiological factors are reduction in renal blood flow during CPB, the mediators generated by the systemic inflammatory response syndrome (SIRS) accompanying CPB and the translocation of endotoxins from the gastrointestinal tract.

Under normal circumstances blood flow to the kidney remains constant despite variations in blood pressure in the range from 80 to 200 mmHg; the kidney thus autoregulates its blood supply. The kidney receives approximately 20% of the total cardiac output (about 1 l/minute). Oxygen delivery thus exceeds 80 ml/minute/100 g tissue. The distribution of blood flow within the kidney is not uniform, with the cortex receiving more than 90% of total blood flow.

Oxygen consumption, however, is less than 10% of total body utilization, and thus there is a low arterio-venous oxygen content difference (1.5 ml oxygen per 100 ml blood). The low oxygen extraction by the kidney suggests that supply exceeds demand and that there should be an adequate oxygen reserve. However, the kidney is highly sensitive to reduction in perfusion, with AKI being a frequent complication of hypotension. The sensitivity of the kidney to damage as a result of hypoperfusion, despite its low overall oxygen consumption, is related to the physiological gradient of intrarenal oxygenation. Within the kidney the cortex and medulla have widely disparate blood flows and patterns of oxygen extraction.

Although a high percentage of blood goes to the cortex (about 5 ml/minute/g), the cortex extracts only about 18% of total oxygen delivered to it. On the other hand, the medullary region has a far smaller blood flow (0.03 ml/minute/g), but has a far greater extraction (about 79% of the delivered oxygen) as a result of the high oxygen requirement for tubular reabsorption of sodium and chloride ions.

Medullary oxygenation is normally strictly balanced by a series of control mechanisms, which match regional oxygen supply and consumption. Failure of these controls renders the outer medullary region susceptible to acute or repeated episodes of hypoxic injury, which may lead to acute tubular necrosis (ATN).

## Hypoxia and renal damage

The differing requirements of cortex and medulla for blood flow and oxygen result in an oxygen tension in the cortex of about 50 mmHg higher than that of the inner medulla. This explains why renal tubules are extremely vulnerable to hypoxic injury and why ATN can be induced by as little as a 40–50% decrease in renal blood flow.

## SIRS and endotoxins

Many of the inflammatory mediators generated by the SIRS associated with CPB are potentially damaging to the kidney. Injury by these mediators results from direct cellular effects, their ability to directly cause vasoconstriction and so impair blood flow, and by their effects on endothelial function in general. For example, during CPB the production of nitric oxide, a smooth muscle relaxant produced by endothelial cells, is reduced and the production of endothelin-1, a potent vasoconstrictor, is increased.

Whilst endotoxins may be directly nephrotoxic, the associated inflammatory responses to circulating endotoxins, in particular the generation of the proinflammatory cytokines such as TNF, mediate further renal damage.

## Prevention of acute kidney injury

General measures that have been proven to prevent AKI include adequate preoperative hydration, avoidance of nephrotoxins (particularly radiocontrast dye) and optimization of hemodynamic parameters.

Unfortunately, pharmacological interventions as a whole have been disappointing in their ability to prevent AKI. Diuretics, including loop and mannitol types, have been evaluated in multiple trials. Most of these have not been controlled, or randomized. Treatment with diuretics is often initiated in response to decrease in urinary flow or clinical signs of volume overload; these situations may be harbingers of/or associated with AKI, but may also be due to decreased effective circulating volume, poor cardiac output or, rarely, urinary tract obstruction. Clearly, diuretics would not be expected to be successful therapeutic interventions specifically for AKI in these situations. Electrolyte imbalance, metabolic alkalosis and renal tubular damage are all associated with diuretic use, leading to concerns about increasing clinical risk with their use.

Studies that have evaluated preoperative use of loop diuretics have shown no benefit in their ability to prevent, correct or shorten the duration of AKI. A non-randomized trial of immediate postoperative utilization of a "cocktail" of mannitol and furosemide compared to furosemide alone among patients deemed high risk for AKI (creatinine >2 mg/dl) demonstrated a 50% decrease in risk of permanent dialysis. However, this study did not control for severity of illness, perioperative events, IABP use or administration of vasopressor drugs. Small series have suggested a benefit from utilization of mannitol in the pediatric population at a dose of 0.5 g/kg body weight. It has been proposed that this is due to mannitol's non-diuretic "free radical scavenger" effect.

Dopamine, utilized at its "renal dose" of 1–3 µg/kg/minute, has long been widely accepted as an agent for prevention and treatment of AKI. However, recent randomized trials have disproven its benefit. Whether it may have a role in truly diuretic-resistant situations of volume overload due to its proximal renal tubular natriuretic effects remains controversial.

Fenoldapam is a more specific dopaminergic agent that has been proposed as an alternative to dopamine. Unfortunately, a controlled trial among patients with chronic kidney disease (CKD) undergoing CABG receiving presurgical angiography showed that the agent failed to prevent AKI, nor did its use reduce 30-day mortality, dialysis requirements or decrease rehospitalization rates.

N-acetylcysteine has shown some promise in trials with respect to its ability to prevent radiocontrast nephrotoxicity. However, a randomized, controlled trial of approximately 300 CKD patients undergoing CABG at high risk for AKI revealed no benefit of N-acetylcysteine.

Natriuretic peptides are also theoretically attractive as agents for the prevention of AKI. Synthetic atrial natriuretic peptide (ANP), anaritide and a synthetic brain natriuretic peptide, neseritide, have been studied in the context of AKI and congestive heart failure. The ability of these agents to prevent AKI, decrease mortality rates and lessen the clinical severity of AKI in multiple models (sepsis, ischemia, toxin exposure) has been demonstrated in animals. Unfortunately, a randomized, double-blind controlled human trial of patients undergoing CABG with or without mitral valve repair showed no clinically meaningful benefit. Natriuretic peptides have also failed to prevent AKI among patients with congestive heart failure.

Theophylline, dexamethasone, pentoxyphyline, clonidine and diltiazem have also been evaluated as preventative agents. Unfortunately, none of these agents proved superior to standard care/placebo therapy with respect to prevention of AKI.

Finally, prophylactic dialysis has been proposed for patients with pre-existing advanced kidney disease. Mortality and prolonged requirement for dialysis was studied among a very small, non-controlled cohort of patients treated with prophylactic dialysis (serum creatinine preoperatively greater than 2.5 mg/dl). Mortality decreased from 30% to 5% and 30-day dialysis requirement was less common in the interventional arm. This controversial approach has yet to be duplicated/replicated.

## Management of dialysis-dependent patients

Patients with CKD who are already dialysis dependent on presentation for cardiac surgery should be dialysed close to the time of operation, generally this is best done in the 1–2 days preceding surgery, to optimize their metabolic and circulatory volume status. Arrangements should also be made for dialysis to re-commence in the early postoperative period. These patients may benefit from intraoperative hemofiltration/ultrafiltration while on CPB to maintain acid–base and electrolytes within normal limits, particularly to remove the potassium load imposed by cardioplegia administration. Hemofiltration/ultrafiltration may be required in the immediate postoperative period to manage fluid balance as well as biochemical parameters.

In the immediate postoperative period, hemofiltration/ultrafiltration provides a temporizing measure in these patients until they are sufficiently stable to be re-established on their usual dialysis regimen.

## Management of patients with non-dialysis-dependent CKD

Patients with evidence of chronic renal impairment, but who do not have sufficiently advanced renal disease to warrant dialysis, may benefit from intraoperative hemofiltration/ultrafiltration while on CPB to optimize acid–base and electrolyte status during surgery. Such patients, as discussed above, have a high likelihood of developing AKI in the postoperative period and may require renal replacement therapy postoperatively until their renal function returns to a viable level.

## Therapy for AKI

Supportive therapy for AKI includes avoidance of further nephrotoxins and optimization of ventilation, perfusion and hemodynamic parameters. Timely management of acid–base and electrolyte abnormalities and ensuring the adequacy of circulating volume are priorities.

# Hyperkalemia

Hyperkalemia commonly complicates AKI and may be immediately life threatening. Emergency treatment of hyperkalemia includes the myocyte membrane-stabilizing effects of calcium chloride or gluconate initially, followed by attempts to shift potassium from the extracellular space to the intracellular space. Infusion of insulin and dextrose, administration of bicarbonate and perhaps the utilization of beta agonists are first-line approaches. Enhanced renal excretion of potassium in AKI may be facilitated by loop diuretics after assurance of adequate intravascular volume. Administration of colonic binding resins such as polystyrene sulfonate by enema or orally with sorbitol has historically been an accepted clinical practice. Recently, documented cases of colonic necrosis associated with the use of binding resins, as well as lack of relative clinical efficacy, has dampened enthusiasm for its use. Failure of these measures to correct hyperkalemia, or its presence accompanying oliguria, require the institution of dialysis.

The metabolic acidosis associated with AKI is commonly due to decreased tissue perfusion and consequent lactic acidosis. Treatment of the underlying pathophysiology is the preferred therapy. The acidosis associated with AKI may initially be exacerbated by accumulation of phosphates, sulfates and other organic anions. Severe acidemia (pH <7.1) may derange adrenergic receptor function, promote pulmonary vasoconstriction and dramatically increase minute ventilation requirements. Therapy specifically to correct severe acidemia using sodium bicarbonate may thus be justified. Dialysis supplies massive amounts of bicarbonate via conductive means, i.e., transfer across the dialysis membrane, and is an extremely efficient means of supplementing bicarbonate without sodium and volume overload.

# Hyponatremia and hypernatremia

Management of hypo- or hypernatremia becomes nearly impossible without adequate renal function. Severe dysnatremia with associated encephalopathy may require dialytic therapy when complicating oliguric AKI. The rate of correction of plasma sodium disturbance needs to be carefully considered, and often continuous dialysis modalities may be best. When medical management fails and/or volume overload occurs, dialysis/extracorporeal renal replacement therapy may be required.

# Oliguria

Use of high-dose diuretics has been advocated by some to convert oliguric to non-oliguric renal failure. In general, these strategies have not been found to decrease mortality, hospitalization or requirements for long-term dialysis. In fact, patients treated with diuretics who are successfully converted from oliguric to non-oliguric renal failure, but who subsequently go on to require dialysis, have increased mortality risk as opposed to oliguric patients started on dialysis within the first 48 hours of nephrology consultation. This calls into question the "automatic" use of diuretics in oliguric AKI, an important shift in common clinical practice. Whether "resting the kidney" occurs with the use of loop diuretics remains controversial. Evaluation of effective circulating volume is critical in AKI, and use of diuretics without clinical signs of volume overload should be questioned.

# Renal replacement therapy

Renal replacement therapy is generally recommended when volume status cannot be medically managed and severe metabolic derangements are manifest (including hyperkalemia, severe hyper- or hyponatremia and severe metabolic acidosis). Additionally, severe azotemia/ uremia may be a relative indication for initiation of renal replacement therapy. Relative indications for initiation of dialysis, with respect to complicated azotemia, include pericardial effusion, pleural rub, bleeding issues (uremic platelet defect) and encephalopathy, which cannot be absolutely attributed to other etiologies. A BUN level of >100 mg/dl has been clinically adopted as a point at which dialysis should be strongly entertained. The evidence to support this practice is, however, not terribly rigorous by modern standards, and needs to be interpreted within the overall clinical context.

Timing of initiation of renal replacement therapy (continuous or intermittent) remains somewhat empirical. Many experts recommend early intervention, citing decreased requirements for long-term dialysis and more rapid correction of azotemia/uremia and metabolic derangements as sound rationale. However, accounting for whether improvement is the result of early intervention with renal replacement therapy, or would have occurred spontaneously with simpler supportive measures, becomes much more difficult as dialytic modalities are initiated early in the clinical course of AKI.

The choice of intermittent versus continuous renal replacement modalities remains very controversial. Hypothetically, continuous renal replacement therapy, which allows for "online" volume management, solute control, potential management of "cytokinemia" and easier titration of vasopressors, seems intuitively to be a better choice. However, randomized trials have failed to demonstrate a benefit of continuous renal replacement therapy over intermittent hemodialysis among all critically ill patients, particularly among those post cardiovascular surgery.

## Conclusion

AKI complicating cardiovascular surgery portends a grave outcome both acutely and in the long term. As non-remediable demography and pre-existing illnesses play such a large role in the development of intra- and perioperative kidney injury, appropriate preoperative counseling of patients and their families regarding these risks is critically important. All efforts should be undertaken to prevent adverse outcomes by maximizing general supportive measures and specifically avoiding nephrotoxins. Prompt initiation of medical and extracorporeal therapy, coordination of care among the multiple care teams and avoidance of further iatrogenic complications will maximize positive outcomes among these high-risk patients.

## Suggested Further Reading

- Adabag AS, Ishani A, Koneswaran S, et al. Utility of N-acetylcysteine to prevent acute kidney injury after cardiac surgery: a randomized controlled trial. Am Heart J 2008; **155**(6): 1143–9.

- Brown JR, Cochran RP, Dacey LJ, et al. Northern New England Cardiovascular Disease Study Group. Perioperative increases in serum creatinine are predictive of increased 90-day mortality after coronary artery bypass graft surgery. Circulation 2006; **114**(1 Suppl): I409–13.

- Chertow GM, Levy EM, Hammermeister KE, Grover F, Daley J. Independent association between acute renal failure and mortality following cardiac surgery. Am J Med 1998; **104**(4): 343–8.

- Hilberman M, Myers BD, Carrie BJ, Derby G, Jamison RL, Stinson EB. Acute renal failure following cardiac surgery. J Thorac Cardiovasc Surg 1979; 77(6): 880–8.

- Hix JK, Thakar CV, Katz EM, Yared JP, Sabik J, Paganini EP. Effect of off-pump coronary artery bypass graft surgery on postoperative acute kidney injury and mortality. *Crit Care Med* 2006; **34**(12): 2979–83.

- Lassnigg A, Donner E, Grubhofer G, Presterl E, Druml W, Hiesmayr M. Lack of renoprotective effects of dopamine and furosemide during cardiac surgery. *J Am Soc Nephrol* 2000; **11**(1):97–104.

- Lombardi R, Ferreiro A, Servetto C. Renal function after cardiac surgery: adverse effect of furosemide. *Renal Failure* 2003; **25**(5): 775–86.

- Ranucci M, Ballotta A, Kunkl A, *et al.* Influence of the timing of cardiac catheterization and the amount of contrast media on acute renal failure after cardiac surgery. *Am J Cardiol* 2008; **101**(8): 1112–8.

- Rosner MH, Okusa MD. Acute kidney injury associated with cardiac surgery. *Clin J Am Soc Nephrol CJASN* 2006; **1**(1): 19–32.

- Schetz M, Bove T, Morelli A, Mankad S, Ronco C, Kellum JA. Prevention of cardiac surgery-associated acute kidney injury. *Int J Artificial Org* 2008; **31**(2): 179–89.

- Sirivella S. Gielchinsky I. Parsonnet V. Mannitol, furosemide, and dopamine infusion in postoperative renal failure complicating cardiac surgery. *Ann Thorac Surg* 2000; **69**(2): 501–6.

- Smith MN, Best D, Sheppard SV, Smith DC. The effect of mannitol on renal function after cardiopulmonary bypass in patients with established renal dysfunction. *Anaesthesia* 2008; **63**(7): 701–4.

- Thakar CV, Worley S, Arrigain S, Yared JP, Paganini EP. Influence of renal dysfunction on mortality after cardiac surgery: modifying effect of preoperative renal function. *Kidney Int* 2005; **67**(3): 1112–9.

# Chapter 7

# Extracorporeal membrane oxygenation

Ashish A. Bartakke and Giles J. Peek

Extracorporeal Membrane Oxygenation (ECMO) enables the technology associated with cardiopulmonary bypass to be utilized in the setting of intensive care units. Although ECMO is based on CPB there are fundamental differences (see Table 14.1).

ECMO provides a means of supporting blood gas exchange using a membrane oxygenator. Venous blood is pumped through the oxygenator, where gas exchange occurs, and is actively re-warmed before being returned to the patient, via either the venous or arterial circulation. There are thus two types of ECMO (see Table 14.2):

- **veno-venous (VV) ECMO**, in which blood is returned to the patient via a vein; and
- **veno-arterial (VA) ECMO**, in which the blood is returned to an artery.

VA ECMO provides gas exchange as well as direct cardiac support, as arterial circulatory flow is augmented by the pump in the ECMO circuit. VV ECMO only provides gas exchange.

## History

The first successful use of ECMO was reported by Hill for the treatment of posttraumatic ARDS in an adult patient in 1972. Following this early success, in 1979 Zapol conducted a randomized controlled trial of VA ECMO in adult patients in the USA. It showed no benefit of VA ECMO compared to continued conventional treatment with approximately 10% survival in each group. However, this trial was fundamental to the development of a number of treatment principles relating to ECMO:

- selecting patients before irreversible ventilator-associated lung injury has occurred;
- the use of lung protective ventilation;
- the use of low-range heparinization; and
- the use of veno-venous ECMO for respiratory support.

Following Zapol's study, clinical ECMO use was largely confined to indications in the neonatal and pediatric age groups. Field and coworkers (Bennett *et al.* 2001) proved that ECMO improves survival in neonates with severe respiratory failure (UK Collaborative ECMO Trial Group) confirming the earlier work (Bartlett *et al.* 1985; O'Rourke *et al.* 1989). The use of ECMO for the treatment of adult patients was taken up again in the late 1980s by a number of groups using the lessons learnt from Zapol's study and neonatal ECMO.

## Indications

Because ECMO can potentially take over the function of both heart and lungs, it can be used for the management of both cardiac and respiratory conditions. Veno-venous ECMO is usually used to support patients with respiratory dysfunction, whereas VA ECMO may be utilized

*Cardiopulmonary Bypass*, ed. S. Ghosh, F. Falter and D. J. Cook. Published by Cambridge University Press.
© Cambridge University Press 2009.

**Table 14.1.** Differences between CPB and ECMO

|  | CPB | VA ECMO |
| --- | --- | --- |
| Setup | Operating room | Intensive care unit |
| Circuit: |  |  |
| Venous reservoir | Yes | No |
| Arterial filter | Yes | No |
| Heparin dose | High | Low |
| ACT levels | >400 seconds | 160–180 seconds |
| Hypothermia | Yes/No | No |
| Anemia | Yes | No |
| Cardiac arrest induced | Yes/No | No |

**Table 14.2.** Differences between veno-arterial and veno-venous ECMO

|  | Veno-arterial ECMO | Veno-venous ECMO |
| --- | --- | --- |
| Cannulation site | Vein: | Vein: |
|  | – internal jugular, | – internal jugular vein |
|  | –femoral | –femoral vein |
|  | –right atrium | –saphenous veins |
|  | Artery: | –right atrium |
|  | –right common carotid |  |
|  | –femoral |  |
|  | –aorta |  |
| Systemic perfusion | Circuit flow and cardiac output | Cardiac output |
| Circulatory support | Partial to complete | No direct effect |
| Cardiac effects | –Preload ↓, | No significant cardiac effects |
|  | –Afterload ↑, |  |
|  | –Pulse pressure ↓ |  |
| Oxygen delivery capacity | High | Moderate |
| CVP monitoring | Unreliable | Reliable |
| Arterial $P_aO_2$ | Unreliable | Reliable |
| Indices of adequacy of perfusion | –$S_vO_2$ | –arterial blood gas, |
|  | –lactate levels | –lactate levels |
| Recirculation | No | Yes |
| Decrease in ventilator "rest settings" | Rapid | Slow |

to manage severe cardiac dysfunction with associated impairment of blood gas exchange. The main indications for ECMO are summarized in Table 14.3.

# Respiratory ECMO in adults

The current practice of ECMO for adults was pioneered by Bartlett and coworkers in 1988 at the University of Michigan, Ann Arbor. It is based on careful patient selection, the use of

**Table 14.3.** Indications for ECMO

| Neonatal and pediatric | Adult |
|---|---|
| *Respiratory* | |
| • Meconium aspiration syndrome | • Severe pneumonia |
| • Persistent pulmonary hypertension of the newborn | • ARDS |
| • Congenital diaphragmatic hernia | • Severe bronchial asthma |
| • Severe pneumonia | • Thoracic trauma involving lung contusion |
| | • Smoke inhalation injury |
| *Cardiac* | |
| • Cardiac arrest | • Resuscitation: |
| • Failure to wean from cardiopulmonary bypass | –cardiac arrest |
| • Treatment of fulminant myocarditis | –cardiogenic shock |
| | –cardiac trauma |
| | –drug overdose |
| | –hypothermia |
| | –pulmonary edema |
| | –pulmonary embolism |
| | –status asthmaticus |
| | –smoke inhalation |
| | • Procedural support: |
| | –abdominal aortic graft replacement |
| | –angioplasty |
| | –arrhythmia ablation |
| | –tracheal surgery |
| | –cerebral arterio-venous malformation resection |
| | –donor organ preservation |
| | –pulmonary embolectomy |
| | –ventricular assist device placement |

VV ECMO for $CO_2$ removal and oxygenation, and a lung protective ventilatory strategy in order to "rest" the lungs and provide optimal conditions for recovery of lung function. The following criteria determine a patient's suitability for adult ECMO:

• Potential reversibility of the disease – only patients with acute and potentially reversible processes are candidates for ECMO support. Chronic and irreversible pathology, such as malignancy, systemic or interstitial diseases affecting the lungs, are not suitable for management with ECMO.

• Premorbid condition of the patient – even if a disease process may be reversible, in a moribund patient the risks of ECMO are likely to outweigh the benefits.

• Etiology of respiratory failure.

• Duration of ventilation – prolonged ventilation with high airway pressures and/or high inspired oxygen concentrations ($FiO_2$) may pose a contraindication to ECMO as the likelihood of ventilator-induced lung injury (VILI) becoming irreversible increases with the duration of mechanical ventilation.

## Cardiac ECMO in adults

Cardiac arrest and shock are the most common indications for cardiac ECMO support in adults. Survival rates with conventional cardiopulmonary resuscitation (CPR) are <5% in cardiac arrests sustained outside a hospital and 5–15% for cardiac arrests within a hospital. Furthermore, patients requiring CPR for more than 30 minutes have a lower incidence of survival, even if resuscitated within a hospital. Cardiac ECMO, usually conducted as VA ECMO, involves passive drainage of blood via the venous cannula, which is then pumped through the oxygenator into the arterial circulation. With VA ECMO survival may be increased to 30–40%, particularly when:

- patients have some return of spontaneous cardiac output; and
- ECMO can be instituted within 30–60 minutes.

VA ECMO is also used as mechanical circulatory support in patients who fail to wean from cardiopulmonary bypass to allow the heart time to recover after cardiac surgery. The advantages are provision of biventricular and pulmonary support and reduced cost compared to ventricular assist devices (VAD) implantation.

A proportion of patients will not recover sufficient cardiac function to be successfully weaned from ECMO. If appropriate, these patients can be supported with VADs and be bridged to either recovery or transplantation (see also Chapter 9).

## ECMO circuit

The basic ECMO circuit, as shown in Figure 14.1a–c, consists of:

- one or more draining (venous) cannulae;
- plastic tubing;
- a centrifugal or roller pump;
- an oxygenator with gas supplies;
- a heat exchanger; and
- an arterial cannula.

Blood flows via the venous cannula(e) to the pump, which pumps it through the oxygenator where gas exchange takes place. A servo-regulation device may be incorporated in the circuit to limit pump flow speed in the event of reduction in venous drainage. Many oxygenators have an integral heat exchanger to re-warm the blood. From the oxygenator the blood is returned to the patient, either into a large vein – VV ECMO – or an artery – VA ECMO. It is notable that in contrast to most cardiopulmonary bypass circuits the ECMO circuit is "closed," lacking a reservoir. This has important implications for patient management. In a closed system, flow is dependent on venous return to the circuit at all times and related to circulating volume and vascular resistance; consequently there is no reserve volume that can be used to buffer changes in circulatory conditions.

- **Cannulae** – Blood flow in the ECMO circuit is dependent on the size of the cannula. It is directly proportional to the fourth power of the internal diameter of the cannula and inversely proportional to the length of the cannula. Thus, a shorter cannula with a greater internal diameter will provide higher flows through the ECMO circuit.

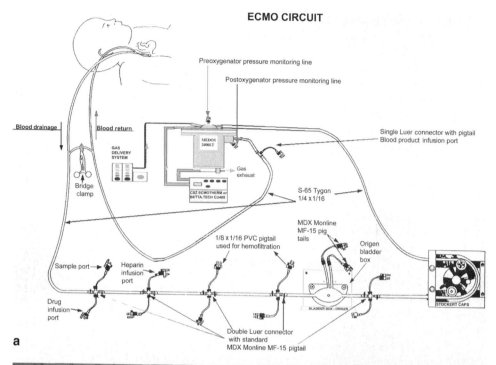

a

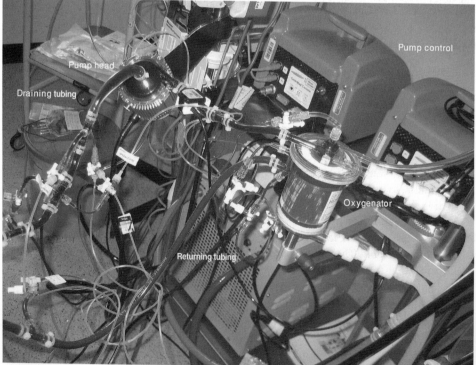

b

**Figure 14.1** (a) Diagram of ECMO circuit; (b) ECMO circuit; (c) patient (prone) supported on VV ECMO.

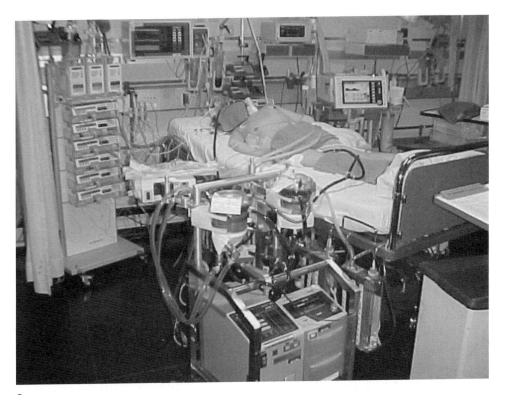

**C**

**Figure 14.1** *Continued.*

Cannulae are usually sized in French gauge (F), which is the circumference of the cannula in millimeters. Typical sizes for adults are:

- arterial : 17–21 F
- venous: 21–28 F
- double lumen venous: 27–31 F

- **Tubing** – This is usually made of PVC or silicon. If a roller pump is used (see below) special super-durable tubing must be used in the raceway to prevent tubing rupture. For adults, tubes of ½ inch internal diameter are used in the drainage line, $^3/_8$ inch or ½ inch in the remainder of the circuit, according to institutional preference. The tubing length is kept as short as possible to reduce surface area and priming volume.

- **Pump** – The pump is the heart of the ECMO circuit. There are two types of pumps currently available. These are the centrifugal pump and the roller pump:

  - Centrifugal pumps – These utilize the spinning action of cones to create a constrained vortex, like a tornado, sucking blood into the pump head and expelling it from its outer edge. Centrifugal pumps must be used with venous line pressure monitoring to prevent excessive negative pressure and hemolysis. CentriMag (Levitronix), RotaFlow (Maquet) and BioConsole 550 (Medtronic Perfusion) are examples of centrifugal pumps commonly used for ECMO.

  - Roller pumps – These are positive displacement devices that compress the plastic tubing and physically push blood forwards. Venous drainage is passive and can be assisted by raising the height of the patient's bed above the ECMO base. Roller pumps must be used with a servo-regulation device, such as a bladder box (OriGen), Stockert pressure servo-regulator (SIII) or the Better-Bladder (CTI), otherwise dangerously excessive negative pressure and cavitation can occur. Any air entering the circuit or generated in the circuit as a result of cavitation may be pumped into the patient. Because the risk of air entrainment is far greater with roller than centrifugal pumps, centrifugal pumps are preferred for ECMO by most institutions.

- **Oxygenators** – These are more correctly termed "membrane lungs" as their function is gas exchange. Three types of oxygenators are commonly used:
  - silicone spiral coil oxygenators;
  - polypropylene oxygenators; and
  - poly-methyl pentene (PMP) oxygenators.

The original silicone spiral coil oxygenator (Medtronic) has been largely superseded by PMP hollow fiber oxygenators (Medos, Maquet & Dideco). They have a lower resistance, lower priming volume and are more biocompatible. PMP oxygenators do not develop the plasma leak seen with polypropylene devices.

- **Heat exchanger** – This warms the blood before it is returned to the heart, thus allowing patient temperature regulation through the ECMO circuit. Most adult oxygenators have an integral heat exchanger.
- **Bridge** – This is a connecting channel between the arterial and venous limbs of the circuit. It is used as a bypass when it is necessary to isolate the patient from the circuit, i.e., blood can be re-circulated within the ECMO circuit in order to prevent stagnation and coagulation. Isolation of the patient from the circuit may be required during circuit maintenance, or during a trial of weaning from VA ECMO. When not in use the bridge is either not inserted (preferable) or kept clamped and flushed every 10–15 minutes.
- **Monitoring and safety devices** – Ultrasonic flow measurement devices are placed around the ECMO circuit tubing and alarm limits are set to warn of low or high flows. Drainage line pressure monitors are used to measure pressure in the venous draining cannula, which is usually negative. When the line pressure becomes very negative (i.e., more than –70 mmHg in an adult), it can cause a non-wire wound cannula to collapse and cause hemolysis. Increasingly, negative venous line pressure may indicate hypovolemia or mechanical obstruction, for example if the tip of the cannula abuts against the vessel wall, leading to occlusion. Line pressure is also measured on the inflow and outflow from the oxygenator to indicate oxygenator resistance. This may rise if clots are collecting or developing in the oxygenator.

Blood gas analysis may be performed either by in-line monitoring or by intermittent sampling:

- In patients on VA ECMO venous line blood gas samples approximate to mixed venous ($SVO_2$) blood samples and are used to assess the adequacy of extracorporeal support. A $SVO_2$ <65% means that oxygen delivery to the patient is marginal and should be increased by turning up the ECMO circuit flow rate if possible. Postoxygenator blood gas samples taken from the oxygenator outflow indicate the functional status of the oxygenator: low $PO_2$ values imply a poorly functioning oxygenator that needs to be changed.
- During VV ECMO the arterial blood gas is used to adjust the level of support. A reduced $P_aO_2$ (<6 kPa) prompts an increase in blood flow and a raised $P_aCO_2$ (>6 kPa) prompts an increase in sweep gas flow.

- **Anticoagulation** – Activated clotting time (ACT) analyzers are an important part of the ECMO monitoring equipment. ACT is usually maintained in the 160–180 seconds range and the rate of heparin infusion is titrated accordingly. This range ensures prevention of clotting within the circuit without causing excessive bleeding. Thromboelastography (TEG) may also be useful for monitoring anticoagulation during ECMO.

## Inflammatory response to ECMO

The circuit tubing and oxygenator are primarily responsible for the inflammatory response that is observed after putting patients on ECMO, as is evidenced by worsening of the chest X-ray following initiation of ECMO. The inflammatory response may be reduced by using albumin to coat the circuit during priming. The use of polymethyl pentene membrane oxygenators has further reduced the inflammatory response. Coating of the oxygenator membrane with heparin may also contribute to the reduction in the inflammatory and coagulative response. A variety of commercial circuit coatings exist – these may be heparin or non-heparin based. Other measures to reduce the inflammatory response may include the use of steroids and hypothermia.

## Cannulation

- **Veno-venous** – Cannulae used for VV ECMO are either single or double lumen. Cannulation sites for single lumen cannulae include the right or left internal jugular vein, or the right or left femoral veins. The right internal jugular vein is used for cannulation with a double lumen cannula. The double lumen cannula is placed in such a way that the distal end of the cannula is in the inferior vena cava, the proximal drainage port is in the superior vena cava and the re-infusion port is in the low right atrium directed at the tricuspid valve. Cannulation is a percutaneous procedure performed under full surgical asepsis. Preventing air embolism is essential. Prophylactic antibiotics are given. Heparin 50–100 U/kg is administered prior to cannulation. For larger patients (weight >90 kg) additional drainage cannulae may be used to ensure adequate flows. The position of the cannulae is confirmed by a plain chest X-ray.
- **Veno-arterial** – In addition to single lumen venous cannulation as described above, an artery is instrumented. The femoral artery is the usual site in adults due to its ease of access. Cannulation will typically be percutaneously; however, in some cases an open dissection may become necessary to place the cannula under direct vision. If the cannulated leg becomes ischemic, distal perfusion must be restored either by moving the cannula or by inserting an antegrade or retrograde distal perfusion cannula.

## Management

Prior to accepting a patient for ECMO a detailed medical history should be obtained. Ideally, a discussion of the patient's current condition and any comorbid disease should take place between members of a multidisciplinary ECMO team. It is helpful to have standardized documentation available for ECMO patients to record observations, results and progress.

An emergency cart, containing items required for cannulation and connection to the ECMO circuit, should also be available. The typical contents of an ECMO cart are listed in Table 14.4.

On arrival of the patient in the accepting ECMO center, baseline investigations, as outlined in Table 14.5, should be performed. Underlying disease, patient condition and institutional protocol may make any number of additional investigations necessary.

**Table 14.4.** Contents of an ECMO cart

- Cable tie-gun
- Sterile scissors
- 500 ml bag of 0.9% sodium chloride
- Rapid access intravenous giving set
- Adult bridge
- 50 ml Luer lock syringe
- Connectors appropriate to tubing used
- Antiseptic (e.g., chlorhexidine) spray
- Tie-straps
- Spare pigtails (three-way taps with 3″ extension tubing – used within the ECMO circuitry mainly as ports for blood sampling, drug injections and infusions)
- High-flow taps
- Sterile gloves
- Antiseptic (e.g., Betadine) solution

**Table 14.5.** Baseline investigations

- Full blood count
- Coagulation profile – platelet count, INR, aPTT ratio, serum fibrinogen
- Liver function tests
- Renal function tests
- Blood sugar
- Infection screening – blood, urine and sputum culture; wound swabs

Once the circuit is established, the day-to-day management of patients on ECMO is generally protocol driven. Specialist ECMO nurses or perfusionists, who can make adjustments or repair the circuit, conduct hourly checks for loose connections, bleeding from cannulation sites and clots within the circuit. They also manage anticoagulation by measuring hourly ACTs to titrate the heparin infusion. A typical infusion dose to maintain adequate anticoagulation is 20–60 IU/kg/hour. Usually the ACT is maintained between 160 and 180 seconds. Blood gases should be monitored continuously or by regular intermittent sampling. Circuit blood flow and sweep gas are adjusted to maintain the desired blood gas parameters.

In addition to careful maintenance of the circuit, the management of the ECMO patient should include:

- **Daily laboratory routine**
  - hematological investigations – full blood count, platelets;
  - biochemistry – urea, electrolytes, creatinine, liver function tests, plasma-free Hb; and
  - coagulation profile – INR, serum fibrinogen, aPTT, APR.
- **Ventilation** – settings should be adjusted to provide lung protective ventilation, i.e.
  - airway pressures should be restricted to <30 cmH$_2$O irrespective of tidal volumes to avoid barotrauma or volutrauma;
  - PEEP of 10–15 cmH$_2$O should be used to prevent further atelectasis;
  - respiratory rate should be limited to 8–10 breaths per minute; and

- FiO$_2$ is reduced to the lowest possible setting to avoid further damage through generation of free oxygen radicals.

If the lungs are "stiff" due to poor compliance, high-frequency oscillatory ventilation (HFOV) can be initiated on ECMO. Ventilation in the prone position has been found to improve gas exchange by allowing adequate aeration of the posterior segments of the lungs. However, turning the ECMO patient should be undertaken with extreme care to avoid dislodgement of ECMO cannulae, other vascular lines and the endotracheal tube.

- **Steroids** – These may be helpful in treating the inflammatory processes during ECMO and ARDS. Methyl prednisolone can be used for this purpose as per the Meduri protocol. A loading dose of 1 mg/kg of methyl prednisolone is administered as a bolus, followed by an infusion of 1 mg/kg from day 1 to day 14, 0.5 mg/kg from day 15 to day 21, 0.25 mg/kg from day 22 to day 25 and 0.125 mg/kg from day 26 to day 28. If the patient is extubated within the first 14 days, they are advanced to day 15 of therapy and then tapered off according to the schedule.
- **Transfusion** – This is a regular occurrence while patients are treated with ECMO. Sepsis, the inflammatory response to foreign surfaces and the mechanical stress caused by ECMO pumps, will cause damage to red blood cells and platelets. In addition anticoagulation may lead to bleeding complications. Blood and platelets are transfused to maintain a platelet count above 80 000 and hematocrit between 40 and 45%. Coagulation is optimized by transfusion of fresh frozen plasma and cryoprecipitate as indicated by clotting study results.
- Nutrition, antibiotic therapy and sedation as well as other daily routine should be managed in accordance with institutional protocols.
- It is advisable to have protocols for other situations, ranging from changing the three-way taps in the circuit to major situations, such as the emergency management of air entrainment into the circuit, in order to ensure these situations are safely handled.

## Weaning and decannulation

Weaning is commenced when the function of the heart and the lungs improve.

- **VV ECMO** – Improvements are seen clinically in lung compliance, chest X-ray appearance and a reduction in the amount of extracorporeal support required. The ECMO flow is gradually reduced; once it is down to approximately 1 l/minute, a "trial off ECMO" can be attempted. This involves increasing the ventilatory support and disconnecting the ECMO sweep gas flow. Following that native gas exchange is assessed by arterial blood gas sampling. Usually, a P$_a$O$_2$ of >8.0 kPa and P$_a$CO$_2$ of 4.5–6.5 kPa during the "trial off ECMO" with lung protective ventilator settings while keeping the FiO$_2$ <60% and respiratory rate <15 breaths/minute indicate sufficiently good gas exchange to allow decannulation.
- **VA ECMO** – Once the heart is deemed to have recovered suitably, flows are reduced and pulse pressure and arterial waveform are assessed. Achieving a mean blood pressure of 60 mmHg without using excessive amounts of inotropes and evidence of adequate tissue perfusion, using indices such as blood gases, acid–base status, serum lactate and S$_v$O$_2$, on 1 l/minute of ECMO flow, is adequate to begin a "trial off ECMO." A 2D echocardiogram is useful to assess the contractility of the heart and any structural and functional cardiac abnormalities. The actual "trial off" proceeds with clamping the patient limb of the ECMO circuit and allowing the blood to circulate through the bridge as described earlier. The patient's response to this maneuver is assessed in terms

of ability to maintain satisfactory cardiovascular parameters and adequate tissue oxygenation. Provided that cardiac function is within acceptable limits on the 2D echocardiogram the patient is decannulated. Percutaneously placed venous cannulae are removed as for VV ECMO using a horizontal mattress suture to close the cannulation site. Decannulation of the artery is usually done by surgical cut-down and usually involves reconstruction of the vessel.

# Conclusion

Extracorporeal membrane oxygenation in adults is an established therapy for treatment of severe respiratory dysfunction where conventional methods are insufficient to treat the patient. The Conventional Ventilation or ECMO for Severe Adult Respiratory Failure (CESAR) trial is a national, randomized, controlled trial conducted in the UK (http://cesar-trial.org), comparing 180 patients treated either with ventilation only or ECMO. The results, when available, will further define the usefulness of ECMO in this situation. The use of cardiac ECMO in adults is very challenging but it is certainly a useful adjunct to the use of VAD and transplantation. ECMO is a complex therapy that is reliant on a skilled multidisciplinary team. As there undoubtedly is a correlation between case load and competence of the team, it is almost always safer to refer the patient to an established ECMO center than to try and extemporize from scratch.

## Suggested Further Reading

- Bartlett RH, Gazzaniga AB, Jefferies MR, Huxtable RF, Haiduc NJ, Fong SW. Extracorporeal membrane oxygenation (ECMO) cardiopulmonary support in infancy. *Trans Am Soc Artif Intern Organs* 1976; **22**: 80–93.

- Bennett C, Johnson A, Field D, Elbourne D. UK collaborative randomised trial of neonatal extracorporeal membrane oxygenation: follow-up to age 4 years. *The Lancet* 2001; **357**(9262): 1094–1096.

- Conventional Ventilation or ECMO for Severe Adult Respiratory Failure. The CESAR Trial. http://cesar-trial.org

- Hill JD, O'Brien TG, Murray JJ, *et al.* Prolonged extracorporeal oxygenation for acute post-traumatic respiratory failure (shock-lung syndrome). Use of the Bramson membrane lung. *N Engl J Med* 1972; **286**: 629–34.

- Khoshbin E, Roberts N, Harvey C, *et al.* Poly-methyl pentene oxygenators have improved gas exchange capability and reduced transfusion requirements in adult extracorporeal membrane oxygenation. *ASAIO J* 2005; **51**(3): 281–7.

- Landis C. Pharmacologic strategies for combating the inflammatory response. *J Extra Corpor Technol* 2007; **39**(4): 291–5.

- Meduri GU, Golden E, Freire AX, *et al.* Methylprednisolone infusion in early severe ARDS: results of a randomized controlled trial. *Chest* 2007; **131**: 954–63.

- Pagani FD, Lynch W, Swaniker F, *et al.* Extracorporeal life support to left ventricular assist device bridge to heart transplant: a strategy to optimize survival and resource utilization. *Circulation* 1999 **100**(19 Suppl.): II206–10.

- Peek GJ, Moore HM, Moore N, Sosnowski AW, Firmin RK. Extracorporeal membrane oxygenation for adult respiratory failure. *Chest* 1997; **112**: 759–64.

- Younger JG, Schreiner RJ, Swaniker F, *et al.* Extracorporeal resuscitation of cardiac arrest. *Acad Emerg Med* 1999; **6**(7): 700–7.

- Zapol WM, Snider MT, Hill JD, *et al.* Extracorporeal membrane oxygenation in severe acute respiratory failure: a randomized prospective study. *JAMA* 1979; **242**: 2193–6.

# Cardiopulmonary bypass in non-cardiac procedures

Sukumaran Nair

Since its first successful use in 1953 by John Gibbon, cardiopulmonary bypass (CPB) has evolved to such an extent that it has become an indispensable tool for cardiac surgeons. The majority of cardiac operations performed use CPB, but CPB can be an essential adjunct in certain non-cardiac procedures. This chapter discusses the various indications to resort to CPB in clinical circumstances outside of the routine cardiac surgical arena.

## CPB in thoracic aortic surgery

Operations on the aorta present a particular challenge because of the unique function of the aorta as the primary conduit for blood flow to the body. Surgical procedures on the aorta can thus only be undertaken by either disrupting flow to some organs completely or by supporting organ perfusion using cardiopulmonary bypass (CPB). Of particular concern are maintenance of blood flow to the brain, kidneys and spinal cord; if blood supply is to be necessarily compromised during the procedure then strategies to protect these organs should be adopted.

Techniques for maintaining effective blood flow to vital organs are dictated by the nature of the underlying pathology and the anatomical site requiring surgical correction.

This chapter summarizes commonly encountered aortic pathology, the surgical approaches used and requirements for perfusion.

The most commonly encountered pathologies are dissection, aneurysmal dilatation and transection of the aorta.

Thoracic aortic disease is classified as follows:

1. **Dissection** – intimal tear/hematoma in media creating a "false" lumen.
2. **Aneurysm** – dilation; atheromatous or associated with Marfan's syndrome.
3. **Transection/tear** – following major trauma.
4. **Coarctation** – congenital narrowing.

## Thoracic aortic dissection

Degeneration of the inner layers of the aortic wall, usually as a result of atheromatous disease, ageing or in association with hypertension, results in a sudden transverse tear of the intima; blood is forced under pressure into a false lumen created by destruction of the substance of the media and stripping of part of the media from the adventitia. Blood flow to organs and limbs may be compromised, depending on the site of the dissection, and the dissection flap may retrogradely extend to the aortic root and/or coronary ostia, giving rise to aortic regurgitation and myocardial ischemia.

Thoracic aortic dissections are classified as per the Stanford classification into:

Type A – involving the ascending aorta; and

Type B – involving the aorta distal to the left subclavian artery.

*Cardiopulmonary Bypass*, ed. S. Ghosh, F. Falter and D. J. Cook. Published by Cambridge University Press.
© Cambridge University Press 2009.

Management is aimed at stopping progression of the dissection. Type A generally requires urgent surgery to limit progression of the dissection into the ascending aorta, prevent aortic regurgitation, intrapericardial rupture and coronary ischemia. Type B is usually managed conservatively using vasodilators and beta blockers.

Type A dissections that do not involve the aortic arch, aortic valve or coronary ostia can be surgically corrected by interposition of a tubular dacron graft to re-establish circulation through the true lumen; stagnation of blood in the false lumen leads to thrombosis and eventually fibrosis. If the aortic valve or coronaries are involved then additionally valve replacement and/or coronary re-vascularization may be necessary. If the aortic arch is involved then more complex surgery is undertaken under deep hypothermic circulatory arrest (DHCA) as discussed later.

In most centers, current surgical practice is to establish CPB, with core cooling, via femoral arterial and venous cannulation before attempting sternotomy. This technique provides "controlled" conditions in the event that the aorta is damaged during chest opening or exposure of the mediastinum; aortic dissections are often associated with fragility and gross anatomical distortion of the mediastinal contents leading to the potential for catastrophic hemorrhage. Commencing cooling early affords protection against neurological damage accompanying sudden, inadvertent hypotension.

Commonly, venous drainage may be poor via the femoral venous cannula; options to improve drainage include using the largest diameter venous cannula that the vein can accommodate, using vacuum-assisted venous drainage, using a long venous cannula that can be passed up the inferior vena cava into the right atrium or placing an additional venous cannula in the right atrium, once the heart has been safely exposed, and connecting the femoral and venous cannula together with a Y-connector to the CPB circuit.

Femoral arterial cannulation may be complicated by the fact that many of these patients also have peripheral vascular disease; cannulation of the vessel may lead to lower limb ischemia. An alternative approach when cannulating peripheral arteries for CPB is to first connect a prosthetic graft, using an end to side anastomosis, to the artery and then placing the cannula in this prosthetic limb rather than directly in the vessel. If the femoral arteries are grossly diseased or too small to accommodate a reasonably sized arterial cannula then the iliac artery may be used instead. A further disadvantage of using the femoral artery for CPB is that perfusion is retrograde and thus, in the face of aortic dissection, may result in blood flowing up the false lumen, compromising rather than improving organ perfusion. At the onset of femoro-femoral CPB particular attention needs to be paid to line pressures, flow rates and the monitored systemic arterial pressure to ensure adequacy of perfusion via the true aortic lumen. The arterial cannula can be transferred to the right axillary artery following sternotomy; this has the advantage of providing antegrade perfusion and may provide better cerebral perfusion than perfusion via the femoral artery. Many surgeons will cannulate the aortic graft as soon as it is in place and use this as the route for arterial return from the CPB machine.

Operative mortality is said to be about 5–10%, with 70% surviving beyond 5 years with good control of hypertension. If the arch is involved then mortality is higher.

# Thoracic aortic aneurysms

Fusiform or saccular dilatation of the aorta as a result of atherosclerosis, cystic medial necrosis or more rarely infection, gives rise to an "aneurysm." The aortic wall in the region of the aneurysm is weakened and prone to rupture, with risk of rupture increasing as the diameter of the aneurysm begins to exceed 5 cm. Aortic aneurysms are classified according to their location into ascending, arch or descending.

1. Ascending – proximal to innominate artery.
2. Arch – between innominate and left subclavian.
3. Descending – distal to left subclavian.

Ascending aneurysms may be treated with an interposition graft, sometimes also requiring aortic valve replacement and coronary ostial re-implantation or coronary bypass grafting. Cannulation for CPB is as described above for aortic dissection.

Arch aneurysms are more complex to correct, requiring replacement of the arch from the innominate artery to the left subclavian artery and anastomosis of the prosthesis to the great vessels. DHCA is required and in addition selective antegrade cerebral perfusion or retrograde cerebral perfusion may be used to try to protect the brain from ischemia. These techniques are discussed in more detail in Chapter 10.

Descending aneurysms require replacement of the aorta from below the left subclavian artery to the diaphragm. A particular hazard is spinal cord ischemia because of the variable origin from the posterior aspect of the aorta of the Radicularis Magna, the principal blood supply of the spinal cord. There are two approaches to descending aortic aneurysm surgery: the older approach is to clamp the aorta proximal to the aneurysm and sew in the graft as rapidly as possible. Alternatively, partial femoro-femoral bypass can be established to maintain perfusion to the lower part of the body. The aorta is clamped proximal and distal to the lesion. Endogenous cardiac output sustains perfusion to the upper half of the body above the proximal aortic clamp. Hypertension in the upper body commonly develops after application of the proximal cross-clamp and needs to be controlled using short-acting vasodilators, or if partial femoral bypass is used by increasing venous drainage into the bypass reservoir and so reducing circulating volume. On completion of the surgical repair, removal of the cross-clamp should be preceded by measures to allow blood pressure and circulating volume to rise, in anticipation of hypotension, and metabolic parameters fully corrected. With regard to the latter, metabolic acidosis is a particular issue following reperfusion of the lower body; if femoral bypass is used a hemofilter can be incorporated in the circuit to assist in metabolic management.

## Reducing spinal cord ischemia during descending aneurysm surgery

As mentioned earlier the blood supply to the spinal cord is particularly vulnerable during descending aortic aneurysm surgery; up to 30% of patients sustain severe neurological injury. The best method of protecting the spinal cord from ischemia is to keep the cross-clamp time short (<30 minutes). Maintaining distal aortic perfusion pressure using partial femoral bypass may help in some cases, but the evidence of significant benefit in preserving neurological function is equivocal. Mild hypothermia may have a role, but again evidence of distinct benefit is lacking. Drainage of cerebrospinal fluid (CSF) to reduce the compression of vessels supplying the spinal cord by rising CSF pressure may be beneficial in maintaining blood flow and is gaining increasing popularity as a protective strategy. Avoidance of hyperglycemia may reduce the damage sustained from ischemia. The role of specific pharmacological agents such as calcium channel blockers remains controversial.

# Blunt thoracic aortic injury

Transection of the aorta occurs as a result of blunt thoracic injury, most commonly road traffic accidents and 80–90% of patients die at the scene. Ninety percent of survivors die within 10 weeks. Survivors have an intact adventitia and the most common site of injury is near the ligamentum arteriosum, distal to the left subclavian artery. Those who reach hospital alive usually have multiple injuries, which may include splenic rupture and head injury. Once adequate assessment and stabilization have been instituted surgical repair of the transection may be appropriate and depends on the site and extent of the tear. Cardiopulmonary bypass may be particularly hazardous because of the need for heparinization in the face of multiple trauma. Use of heparin-bonded circuitry with only partial heparinization has been advocated. Cannulation for CPB depends on the site of the tear and follows the principles discussed above for management of dissections or aneurysms. Use of left heart bypass for emergency aortic repair is described in the section on "CPB in Trauma Care" later in this chapter. With the recent advances made in interventional radiology, percutaneous stenting across the transected aorta has been successfully performed in many instances. Vascular access is achieved through the left common femoral artery and a covered stent is deployed across the transection line under radiological guidance. Long-term performance data of this intervention is awaited.

In conclusion, management of operations on the aorta requires detailed preoperative planning of the choice of initial cannulation site and strategy for improving CPB flow and quality of perfusion with additional cannulation if required, adaptability intraoperatively to resort to DHCA and ability to conduct full or partial CPB. Preoperative "work up" of the patient is crucial, but time may not always be available as many of these procedures are emergent. Intraoperatively key factors in successful outcome are limiting ischemic times, rigorous correction of metabolic parameters and skilled imaging using TOE, not only to define the lesion, but also to assess perfusion within the true lumen of the aorta, valvular competence and cardiac function. Thoracic aortic surgery still carries a high rate of morbidity and mortality.

# Re-warming from severe hypothermia

Every year, approximately 4 out of 1 000 000 people in the USA die as a result of hypothermia. Between 1999 and 2002, 4607 death certificates identified hypothermia or related complications as the underlying cause of death in the USA. Accidental hypothermia is defined as an unintentional decrease in core temperature below 35°C due to hypothermic exposure in individuals without intrinsic thermoregulatory dysfunction. Depending on the degree of core cooling, accidental hypothermia can be mild (32.2–35°C), moderate (28–32.2°C) or deep (below 28°C). Deep accidental hypothermia (DAH) usually follows accidental exposure to extreme cold, resulting in suspension of all signs of life and mimicking death, particularly if an "after drop" in temperature occurs. "After drop" is a phenomenon of conductive heat loss that is usually associated with immersion hypothermia following accidental drowning.

The most important differential diagnosis of severe hypothermia is death. Hyperkalemia may be a useful diagnostic tool to differentiate between these two states. Mair and coworkers in a retrospective study involving 22 hypothermic patients re-warmed with the aid of CPB, suggested that the following were indicative of the inability to restore spontaneous circulation due to irreversible cell death:

- hyperkalemia exceeding 9 mmol/l:
- pH ≤6.5: or
- ACT >400 seconds in a venous blood sample.

Patients with such severely deranged metabolic parameters did not regain spontaneous circulation despite full re-warming on CPB.

Severe hypothermia is a medical emergency. Core re-warming may be required in a short space of time to prevent resistant cardiac arrhythmias and death. There are many ways of re-warming, broadly divided into invasive and non-invasive methods. In the emergency room re-warming techniques are usually limited to administration of warmed intravenous fluids, warming blankets and gastric and bladder lavage. These methods are relatively slow and ineffective. The only reliable way of safely and reliably restoring normothermia relatively quickly is to use CPB.

Other non-invasive techniques for re-warming include:

- warming inspired gases;
- microwave therapy;
- warm water immersion; and
- body cavity lavage, which involves the repeated instillation of up to 2.5l of normal saline into the peritoneal cavity, and leaving it for 20 minutes before draining again – this sequence is repeated until a core temperature of 37°C is achieved.

More recently arterio-venous anastomosis (AVA) warming has been promoted. This involves the application of heat in the form of circulating warm air, with or without negative pressure to distal extremities in an effort to increase AVA blood flow.

In 1996, Kornberger and colleagues published the results of a study where 55 patients who had suffered severe accidental hypothermia were treated using three different methods of re-warming, namely:

- airway re-warming, warmed fluids and insulation in patients in a stable hemodynamic state;
- peritoneal dialysis in patients in an unstable hemodynamic state; and
- extracorporeal circulation in patients who had circulatory arrest.

Survival rates were 100%, 72% and 13%, respectively, in these three groups. This study concluded that the method used to re-warm a patient with severe accidental hypothermia should be adjusted to the hemodynamic status of the patient in order to achieve best results. Prognosis seemed to be excellent in patients with no hypoxic event preceding hypothermia and with non-serious underlying disease.

Whenever possible, re-warming should be attempted with invasive methods. Patients with a cardiac output and systolic pressure over 80 mmHg might benefit from continuous arterio-venous re-warming (CAVR) alone. This entails establishing peripheral arterial and venous access to maintain low flow rates through an extracorporeal circuit incorporating a heat exchanger for re-warming. The commonest route of arterial access is via the femoral artery, while venous access is normally established via the femoral or internal jugular vein. The arterial and venous cannulae can be either introduced percutaneously or after a vascular cut down. Arrested and hemodynamically unstable patients should be treated with full CPB using a circuit incorporating an oxygenator. Formal full-dose heparinization is required. The use of pharmacological means of vasodilatation with agents such as sodium nitroprusside during the re-warming phase of CPB has been shown to improve peripheral re-warming; vasodilators enhance the distribution of blood to peripheral vessels and so help to "even out" the core–peripheral temperature difference.

Controlled studies comparing the efficacy of CPB and alternative warming techniques have not been performed so far. In a literature review published by Vretenar et al. in 1994, it was shown that femoro-femoral bypass was used as a means to re-warm 72% of profoundly hypothermic patients. The overall survival was 60% in this series with 80% of the survivors suffering no long-term organ dysfunction.

## CPB in management of acute respiratory failure

Institution of urgent CPB is of value in patients with sustained respiratory arrest or obstruction in whom endotracheal intubation is not possible. This approach can be life-saving in young patients with treatable pathology such as mediastinal lymphadenopathy due to hematological malignancies causing superior vena caval and tracheal obstruction. Mediastinal tumors can compress major airways to such an extent that the occurrence of even mild supraglottic edema can result in complete airway obstruction. This may occur following minimal handling of the airway during attempted endotracheal intubation, or following upper respiratory tract infections. Initiation of femoro-femoral CPB is the only safe interim procedure prior to controlled tracheotomy to secure an airway. This approach provides a safe solution for airway control when intubation or a surgically created airway is either unsuccessful or too hazardous to attempt.

## Management of acute pulmonary embolism

The majority of cardiothoracic surgeons would agree that pulmonary embolectomy is currently rarely indicated as acute pulmonary embolism can be treated effectively and safely with thrombolytic agents, delivered either intravenously or via a pulmonary artery catheter locally. Emergency cardiopulmonary support by CPB in massive pulmonary thromboembolism can be helpful in increasing the efficiency of thrombolytic agents by establishing circulation. A few instances where institution of percutaneous CPB in patients with acute pulmonary embolism was life-saving have been reported. Cardiopulmonary bypass was of use particularly when cardiogenic shock was evident and helped in the immediate resuscitation and stabilization of cardiopulmonary function, allowing for subsequent successful emergency pulmonary embolectomy. Pulmonary embolectomy can also be achieved by pulmonary arteriotomy and retrograde flushing of the pulmonary circulation via the pulmonary veins after establishment of CPB. With the ubiquitous availability of effective thrombolytic agents, surgical pulmonary embolectomy is an infrequently performed procedure in the current era.

## CPB in single and sequential double lung transplantation

CPB has been frequently used for single and double lung transplantation. Certain transplantation centers have been reluctant to resort to CPB during lung transplantation due to potential side effects, including hemorrhage and triggering of the systemic inflammatory response syndrome (SIRS) associated with CPB, leading to sequestration of neutrophils and platelets in the pulmonary capillary bed, endothelial damage, increased capillary permeability and subsequent pulmonary edema. A study from a major center involving 74 patients over 4 years compared patients who had their lung transplant with or without CPB. It failed to demonstrate any significant difference in the short- or long-term outcome of the grafts between the groups, thereby refuting the argument of the adverse effects of CPB-induced SIRS. Most commonly, however, the decision to establish partial or complete CPB is made after hemodynamic assessment of the patient following occlusion of the pulmonary artery during surgery. Criteria for the establishment of CPB include a mean pulmonary artery pressure of more than 50 mmHg, hypoxia, hypercapnea or hemodynamic instability. Prior to surgery it is also possible to get an indication of the need for CPB support by eliminating ventilation to the operative lung. If the non-operative lung is ineffective for maintaining ventilation on its own, the patient is unlikely to tolerate the period of lung isolation during explant and implant of the operative lung and CPB will be required.

As yet, there are no reliable preoperative predictors for the need for CPB in lung transplantation. In a study involving 109 lung transplant recipients, however, the following parameters:

- preoperative right ventricular ejection fraction <40%,
- a 6-minute walk test result of less than 250 m and
- a drop in arterial oxygen saturation on exercise to <94% on room air

were positive predictive factors for resorting to CPB.

# Extracorporeal circulation in liver transplantation

Occasionally extracorporeal circulation is used to assist liver transplantation. In general terms, extracorporeal circulation provides a means of decompressing the hepatoportal circulation and reducing the risk of bleeding when operating on patients with portal hypertension. It also reduces the risk of post-transplantation renal failure and of intestinal venous congestion with subsequent hepatic dysfunction. The femoral vein is cannulated at the groin for venous return using a standard short venous cannula. The venous blood thus drained is passed through a centrifugal pump to be returned to the systemic venous circulation by cannulae inserted into the internal jugular or subclavian vein. The circuit is constituted of heparin-bonded material and full systemic heparinization is avoided if possible.

Systemic venous return is often impaired by surgical manipulation during both excision of the native liver and implantation of the transplant organ. Employing an extracorporeal perfusion technique allows the portal circulation to be decompressed as well as systemic venous return to be maintained at adequate levels to optimize systemic cardiac output. Furthermore, it allows extravasated blood to be salvaged and returned to the circulation. If portal hypertension persists despite inferior vena cava drainage via the femoral vein, an extra-venous drainage cannula can be inserted directly into the portal vein. It should be noted that the circuit described here is not a cardiopulmonary bypass circuit as it does not include a gas exchanger, there is no arterial cannulation and the cardiac output is maintained by the heart.

# CPB in resection of tumors

The commonest indication to resort to cardiopulmonary bypass is the excision of a liver or renal malignancy growing into the inferior vena cava and occasionally into the right atrium. Selective cannulation and snaring of the venae cavae, along with a generous right atriotomy after establishment of CPB, helps the surgeon to extract tumors extending into the inferior vena cava and right atrium under direct vision (see Figure 15.1). With tumors extending into the right atrium, or in exceptional circumstances even into the pulmonary artery, complete excision of the tumor might require deep hypothermic circulatory arrest DHCA.

Cardiopulmonary bypass permits maintenance of systemic perfusion at a low pressure, cessation of pulmonary artery inflow into the lungs and, if required, drainage of the whole circulating volume into the venous reservoir, thereby allowing total circulatory arrest. The risk of stroke and other neurological complications is minimal if DHCA is employed and does not exceed 30 minutes. Cardiopulmonary bypass thus enables safe resection of vascular tumors and tumors occupying anatomical locations that are difficult to access. The risk of hemorrhage and organ damage is reduced by lowering the systemic pressure on CPB, cooling down

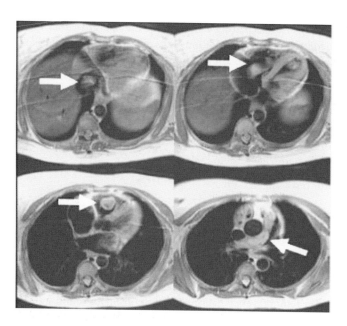

**Figure 15.1** Cardiac-gated MRI scan demonstrating uterine benign leiomyoma extending from pelvis through the inferior vena cava into the right atrium, right ventricle and subsequently into the main pulmonary artery. (Courtesy: Mr Ray George and Mr Jon Anderson, Department of Cardiothoracic Surgery, Hammersmith Hospital.)

the patient and, if required, stopping the circulation completely for a finite period of time to allow surgical dissection in a bloodless field. Mediastinal tumors that are diffuse or infiltrating the heart and great vessels are best excised after institution of CPB. Though infiltration of major vascular structures of the mediastinum can be a contraindication for attempting curative resection of advanced lung cancer, there are studies that have shown a survival benefit when performed in selected patients with advanced T4 lung tumors assisted by CPB.

## CPB in other elective procedures

Resection or decompression of complex arterio-venous malformations of the retroperitoneum, mediastinum, limbs and brain using endovascular embolization with, or without, open surgical techniques will benefit from low-flow CPB or DHCA; CPB and DHCA have been of particular value in converting otherwise inoperable tumors or vascular malformations of the brain or spinal cord to those amenable to a relatively safe surgical procedure.

Profound hypothermia, circulatory arrest and exsanguination is a common approach in certain high-risk neurosurgical interventions to remove intracranial aneurysms, glomus jugulare tumors and hemangioblastoma of the brain. In such instances, DHCA provides a bloodless surgical field and protection of the brain, which make precise clipping of the vascular malformation possible. The disadvantages of this technique include cardiac distension and arrhythmia during CPB, hemorrhage from systemic anticoagulation and central nervous system injury due to inadequate cerebral protection.

## CPB in trauma care

In complex traumatic injuries of intrathoracic organs, institution of CPB can be life-saving. This enables the surgeon to work in a bloodless field with non-ventilated, collapsed lungs. More importantly, CPB ensures that the rest of the body is adequately perfused during the operation and allows salvaging of shed blood.

Aortic injury is the commonest and most serious intrathoracic injury. Total CPB, as mentioned earlier, or at least left heart bypass, should be resorted to before attempting repair of an aortic tear or rupture. The technique of left heart bypass may be used for repair of the descending aorta: after thoracotomy the left atrium is typically cannulated via a pulmonary vein, and oxygenated blood is drained to a pump which is used to return the oxygenated blood via a femoral arterial cannula. This provides perfusion to organs below the distal aortic cross-clamp. The left ventricle is partially decompressed and ejects the remainder of the left atrial volume into the aorta to supply the head and neck vessels. This allows cross-clamping of the injured aorta above and below the site requiring repair or replacement, while circulation is maintained to all vital organs. The lungs continue to function as the means of gas exchange.

CPB is also essential in the emergency repair of multiple or single chamber heart injury. In 1990, Reichman and coworkers published their results of using CPB for the treatment of cardiac arrest after trauma. Of the 38 patients in their series, 95% were successfully resuscitated and 50% weaned from bypass, although the overall survival rate was only 16%. The main reason attributed to account for this poor outcome was the need for full heparinization, which resulted in high rates of bleeding complications. Far better results were reported by Perchinsky and coworkers in 1995 using heparin-bonded circuits. They demonstrated a survival rate of 50% in six patients with severe pulmonary injuries and profuse hemorrhage.

## CPB for emergency cardiopulmonary support (ECPS)

The use of a portable CPB device in the emergency room to resuscitate patients with severe hypothermia or thoracic trauma is controversial. The need for systemic anticoagulation with heparin, and the subsequent bleeding complications in the setting of trauma, generally result in an increased demand for transfusion, which has limited widespread application of the technique. Moreover, initial experience showed disappointing results for trauma patients. The introduction of heparin-bonded circuitry in the ECPS system has improved survival rates.

## Portable ECPS device

The development of a portable ECPS system soon followed the first successful use of CPB. In 1954, its usage was limited to the operating theater and to the field of cardiac surgery. In the 1970s, ECPS became an evolving therapeutic option for treating medical emergencies. In 1972, Hill and coworkers reported the first successful application of extracorporeal membrane oxygenation in a patient with traumatic respiratory failure. Later, cardiologists started using portable ECPS for supporting patients after high-risk angioplasties and other interventional procedures following myocardial infarction.

### Concept of ECPS

The system consists of a pump, an oxygenator, tubing and percutaneous venous and arterial cannulae. Cannula sizes vary from 17 to 19 Fr for the arterial cannula and 19 to 21 Fr size for the venous cannula. The vessels are cannulated either percutaneously or by direct cut down. Full heparinization monitored by serial ACT measurements is required. Blood is drained from a large-bore central vein, usually the femoral vein, and perfused back, after oxygenation, via the femoral artery. A heat exchanger included in the circuit helps to control temperature.

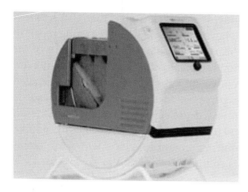

**Figure 15.2** Lifebridge B2T is one of the first fully portable emergency life support systems for patients suffering cardiogenic shock. First introduced in 2005, currently it has a CE mark for use all over Europe. It measures 61 × 45 × 37 cm and weighs 17.5 kg with an ability to generate up to 6 l/minute flow with peripheral or central arterio-venous cannulation.

**Table 15.1.** Main indications for ECPS, National Registry of Cardiopulmonary Support for Emergency Applications

| Indications | Percentage of patients |
|---|---|
| Cardiogenic arrest post cardiotomy | 55 |
| Cardiogenic shock | 9 |
| Cardiogenic shock post cardiotomy | 18 |
| Hypothermia | 5 |
| Pulmonary insufficiency | 6 |
| Others | 7 |

Currently, portable ECPS devices are available commercially for emergency cardiopulmonary support (see Figure 15.2).

The National Registry of Cardiopulmonary Support for Emergency Applications details the main indications for ECPS (see Table 15.1). It reflects the large experience of using ECPS in the operating theater and cardiology catheter laboratories. In this database, 63% of all patients died while on a ECPS system. Ten percent of patients lived for less than 30 days while 25% survived for more than 30 days. Unwitnessed cardiac arrest resulted in a high mortality even after resorting to ECPS.

Though the success of survival in witnessed cardiac arrest patients supported with ECPS was better than in the unwitnessed group, mortality was still over 70%. Patients who survived had more therapeutic procedures undertaken than the non-survivors, suggesting that complete correction of precipitating medical factors is important for a successful outcome. Though severely compromised patients can be resuscitated effectively for a period of up to 6 hours with the ECPS, further therapeutic or diagnostic steps need to be undertaken in order to save the patient's life. While ECPS is not a therapy by itself, it has been proven to buy time, potentially allowing for the correction of underlying disease processes. New heparin-bonded circuitry avoids the need for full dose heparin, thus allowing ECPS to be used in patients with acute hemorrhage or other contraindications for extracorporeal circulation.

Definitive criteria for defining the patients who will benefit most from treatment with ECPS are still lacking, and future research should be directed to provide more information regarding this issue.

# Suggested Further Reading

- Apostolakis E, Akinosoglou K. The methodologies of hypothermic circulatory arrest and of antegrade and retrograde cerebral perfusion for aortic arch surgery. *Ann Thorac Cardiovasc Surg* 2008; **14**(3): 138–48 (Review).

- Centers for Disease Control and Prevention. Hypothermia-related deaths: United States, 1999–2002 and 2005. MMWR 2006; 55: 282–4.

- De Perrot M, Fadel E, Mussot S, De Palma A, Chapelier A, Dartevelle P. Resection of locally advanced (T4) non-small cell lung cancer with cardiopulmonary bypass. *Ann Thorac Surg* 2005; **79**(5): 1691–6.

- Hill JD, O'Brien TG, Murray JJ, *et al.* Prolonged extracorporeal oxygenation for acute post-traumatic respiratory failure (shock-lung syndrome): use of the Bramson membrane lung. *N Engl J Med* 1972; **286**: 629–34.

- Hlozek C, Smedira N, Kirby T, Patel A, Perl M. Cardiopulmonary bypass (CPB) for lung transplantation. *Perfusion* 1997; **12**(3): 107–12.

- Hoyos A, Demajo W, Snell G, *et al.* Preoperative prediction for the use of cardiopulmonary bypass in lung transplantation. *J Thorac Cardiovasc Surg* 1993; **11**(106): 787–95.

- Kornberger E, Mair P. Important aspects in the treatment of severe accidental hypothermia: the Innsbruck experience. *J Neurosurg Anesthesiol* 1996; **8**(1): 83–7.

- Mair P, Kornberger E, Furtwaenglere, Balogh D, Antretter H. Prognostic markers in patients with severe accidental hypothermia and cardiocirculatory arrest. *Resuscitation* 1994; **27**(1): 47–54.

- Patel HJ, Deeb GM. Ascending and arch aorta: pathology, natural history, and treatment. *Circulation* 2008; **118**(2): 188–95 (Review).

- Perchinsky M, Long W, Hill J, Parsons J, Bennett J. Extracorporeal cardiopulmonary life support with heparin-bonded circuitry in the resuscitation of massively injured trauma patients. *Am J Surg* 1995; **169**: 488–91.

- Pocar M, Rossi V, Addis A, *et al.* Spinal cord retrograde perfusion: review of the literature and experimental observations. *J Card Surg* 2007; **22**(2): 124–8 (Review).

- Reichman R, Joyo C, Dembitsky W, *et al.* Improved patient survival after cardiac arrest using a cardiopulmonary support system. *Ann Thorac Surg* 1990; **49**: 99–101.

- Vogel R, Shawl F, Tommaso C, *et al.* Initial report of the National Registry of Elective Cardiopulmonary Bypass Supported Coronary Angioplasty. *J Am Coll Cardiol* 1990; **15**: 23–9.

- Vretenar D, Urschel J, Parrott J, Unruh H. Cardiopulmonary bypass resuscitation for accidental hypothermia. *Ann Thorac Surg* 1994; **58**(9): 895–8.

- Wong DR, Lemaire SA, Coselli JS. Managing dissections of the thoracic aorta. *Am Surg* 2008; **74**(5): 364–80 (Review).

# Index

## A

acid-base management
DHCA, 132–3
acid-base status during CPB, 74–5
acidosis. *See* metabolic acidosis; respiratory acidosis
activated clotting time (ACT), 43, 47, 61
acute ischemia during CPB, 89
acute kidney injury (AKI), 167–74
acute tubular necrosis (ATN), 170
definitions, 167–8
effects of endotoxins, 171
effects of SIRS, 171
etiology, 170–1
hyperkalemia therapy, 173
hypo- and hypernatremia therapy, 173
hypoxia and renal damage, 170
incidence, 167
management of dialysis-dependent patients, 172
management of patients with non-dialysis-dependent CKD, 172
oliguria therapy, 173
outcomes associated with, 168
prevention strategies, 171–2
renal replacement therapy, 173–4
risk factors for, 169–70
therapy for AKI, 172–4
acute pulmonary embolism use of CPB, 192
acute respiratory distress syndrome (ARDS) post-CPB, 150–1
acute respiratory failure use of CPB, 192
acute tubular necrosis (ATN), 170
adrenaline (epinephrine), 103
alarm systems

CPB monitoring, 20
re-enabling before weaning from CPB, 96
albumin, 39
alkalosis
metabolic, 74–5
respiratory, 75
alpha-stat management of blood gas, 75, 132–3
ε-aminocaproic acid (EACA), 50–1, 131
anesthesia
for DHCA, 126–8
weaning from CPB, 95
analgesia
weaning from CPB, 95
antegrade cerebral perfusion (ACP), 74
antegrade delivery of cardioplegia, 84–5
anti-thrombin III (AT-III) deficiency, 43, 61
anticoagulation during CPB, 41–52
activated clotting time (ACT), 47
argatroban, 45
bivalrudin, 45
coagulation cascade, 41
danaproid, 44–5
dangers of clot formation, 41
direct thrombin inhibitors, 45
fibrinolytics, 45
heparin, 42–4
heparin neutralization, 45–7
lepirudin, 45
low-molecular-weight heparin (LMWH), 44
monitoring anticoagulation in the operating room, 47–8
pharmacological strategies, 42–5
point of care (POC) testing, 47–8
transfusion algorithms, 52
anticoagulation reversal, 45–7
weaning from CPB, 94, 101–2

antifibrinolytic agents, 50–1, 131
aorta. *See* thoracic aorta
aortic root replacement
cardioplegia, 89–90
aprotinin, 51, 131
ARDS (acute respiratory distress syndrome)
post-CPB, 150–1
argatroban, 45
arterial blood analysis, 78–9
arterial blood gases
weaning from CPB, 97
arterial cannulae, 3–5
arterial cannulation, 54–7
ascending aorta, 55
axillary artery, 57
cannula types, 54–5
complications of aortic root cannulation, 55–6
connection to the patient, 55
femoral artery, 55–6
innominate artery, 55
performance index of an arterial cannula, 54
peripheral arterial cannulation, 56–7
presence of atherosclerosis, 55
subclavian artery, 55
arterial line filters, 13–4, 23
ascending aorta
arterial cannulation, 3–5
autologous priming of the CPB circuit, 37, 71
AVR surgery, 58

## B

bicarbonate buffer system, 74
bicaval cannulation, 6, 58
bivalrudin, 45
bleeding after CPB
patient management, 51–2
bleeding prevention
ε-aminocaproic acid, 50–1
antifibrinolytic agents, 50–1
aprotinin, 51
desmopressin, 51
heparin dosing, 51

bleeding prevention (*cont.*)
  non-pharmacological
    strategies, 51
  protamine dosing, 51
  tranexamic acid, 50–1
blood-based priming solutions,
  37
blood cardioplegia. *See*
  cardioplegia
blood flow, cessation. *See* deep
  hypothermic circulatory
  arrest (DHCA)
blood gas management
  DHCA, 132–3
  during CPB, 75–6
blunt thoracic aortic injury,
  190–1
brain injury. *See* cerebral
  morbidity in adult cardiac
  surgery
bubble traps and filters,
  13–4
buffer systems, 74

## C

CABG (coronary artery bypass
  graft), 6, 58
  comparison of CPB and
    OPCAB, 151
  *See also* OPCAB.
calcium
  Ca²⁺ electrolyte, 76
  in cardioplegia solutions, 82
carbon dioxide level in the
  patient's blood, 75–6
cardiac function assessment
  weaning from CPB, 95
cardiac surgery
  de-airing the heart, 97
cardioplegia, 80–90
  acute ischemia, 89
  acute MI/arrest cardioplegia,
    89
  alternatives to, 86–7
  antegrade delivery, 84–5
  aortic root replacement,
    89–90
  blood cardioplegia, 82–4
  components of cardioplegia
    solutions, 81–4
  definition, 80
  delivery systems, 84
  evolving myocardial
    infarction, 89
  goals and principles of
    myocardial protection, 81–2

integrated method of
  administration, 87–9
  modifications for particular
    situations, 89–90
  monitoring distribution by
    temperature, 86
  myocardial damage during
    CPB, 80
  optimum cardioplegia
    technique, 87–9
  prevention of septal
    dysfunction, 89
  retrograde delivery, 84–5
  routes of cardioplegia
    delivery, 84–6
  temperature of the
    cardioplegia solution, 86
cardioplegia delivery systems,
  15–7, 23, 84
cardioprotective strategies. *See*
  cardioplegia
cardiopulmonary bypass (CPB)
  definition, 1
  history of development, 1
  modifications for DHCA,
    129–30
  rates of patient injury or
    death, 28
  versus OPCAB, 148
cardiopulmonary bypass circuit
  reducing priming volume, 70
cardiopulmonary bypass circuit
  assembly, 23–8
  approaches to the setup
    procedure, 23–5
  disposable items, 23
  pre-bypass checklist, 25
  priming solutions, 36–40
  review of patient's notes, 25
  safety issues, 23, 25, 28
cardiopulmonary bypass circuit
  primes. *See* priming solutions
  for CPB circuits
cardiopulmonary bypass in
  non-cardiac procedures,
  187–96
  blunt thoracic aortic injury,
    190
  emergency cardiopulmonary
    support (ECPS), 195–6
  liver transplantation, 193
  management of acute
    pulmonary embolism, 192
  management of acute
    respiratory failure, 192
  rewarming from severe
    hypothermia, 190–2

single and double lung
  transplantation, 192–3
  thoracic aortic aneurysms,
    189–90
  thoracic aortic dissection,
    187–8
  thoracic aortic surgery,
    187–90
  trauma care, 194–5
  tumor resection, 193–4
cardiopulmonary bypass
  machine
  basic circuit, 1
cardiopulmonary bypass
  procedure, 54–67
  adequate tissue perfusion,
    62–4
  arterial cannulation, 54–7
  cardiotomy suction, 59
  central venous pressure
    (CVP), 64
  electrocardiogram (ECG), 64
  general management, 61–6
  hemodilution, 63
  hypothermic CPB, 65
  laboratory investigations, 66
  left atrial (LA) pressure, 64
  mean arterial pressure
    (MAP), 63–4
  multidisciplinary approach,
    54
  planning, 54
  pulmonary artery (PA)
    pressure, 64
  recommended flow rates for
    CPB, 62–3
  systemic oxygen delivery
    (DO₂), 62–3
  systemic oxygen demand
    (VO₂), 62–3
  temperature, 65
  termination of CPB, 66–7
  transition of patient onto
    CPB, 61–2
  transesophageal
    echocardiography (TOE),
    65–6
  urine volume, 65
  venous cannulation and
    drainage, 57–8
  venting the heart, 60–1
  weaning from CPB, 66–7
cardiothoracic surgery
  optimal surgical field, 1
cardiotomy reservoir, 8–9
cardiotomy suction, 59
  adverse effects, 59

cavitation in roller pumps, 8
cavitation in venous drainage, 57
cavo-atrial cannulation, 58
central venous pressure (CVP) during CPB, 64
centrifugal pumps, 8
cerebral morbidity in adult cardiac surgery, 153–66
cerebral physiology during CPB, 153–6
determinants of cerebral perfusion, 153–6
effects of glucose control, 157
effects of perfusion pressure, 156
effects of temperature, 156–7
intraoperative ischemia and physiological management, 156–7
neurocognitive outcomes, 163–6
neurological complications, 153
OPCAB and stroke, 159
perioperative stoke, 157–8
risk factors for perioperative stroke, 161–3
stroke and OPCAB, 159
stroke risk in the general population, 161–3
timing of cardiac surgery-related stroke, 159–60
cerebral perfusion during CPB, 153–6
cerebral physiology during CPB, 153–6
cerebral substrate delivery monitoring, 135–6
chest splinting, 105
children
priming solutions for CPB circuits, 36
chloride ions in cardioplegia solutions, 82
chronic kidney disease (CKD), 167, 169, 171
management of dialysis-dependent patients, 172
management of non-dialysis-dependent patients, 172
circulating volume
weaning from CPB, 94
citrate phosphate dextrose (CPD) in cardioplegia solutions, 82, 87

Clot Signature Analyzer, 48
clotting and platelet function assessment
weaning from CPB, 94
coagulation
weaning from CPB, 94
coagulation cascade, 41
activation of the extrinsic pathway, 52
coagulation disorders after CPB, 49–52
antifibrinolytic agents, 50–1
causes, 49–50
effects of hypothermia, 50
fibrinolysis, 50
heparin rebound, 50
management of the bleeding patient, 51–2
platelet abnormalities, 49–50
prevention of bleeding, 50–1
SIRS, 50
Cobe Duo membrane oxygenator, 13
colloid-based priming solutions, 39–40
complement system
role in organ damage during CPB, 143
contact activation, 142–4
coronary artery bypass graft. See CABG
CPB. See cardiopulmonary bypass
CPD in cardioplegia solutions, 82, 87
cross-circulation technique, 1
crystalloid priming solutions, 37–9

**D**

danaparoid, 44–5
deep hypothermic circulatory arrest (DHCA), 55, 73–4, 125–38
acid–base management, 132–3
alpha-stat blood gas management, 132–3
anesthesia, 126–8
applications, 125
blood gas management, 132–3
cerebral substrate delivery monitoring, 135–6
cooling, 129

CPB modifications, 129–30
duration of circulatory arrest, 129
extracorporeal circulation, 129–30
glycemic control, 134
hemodilution, 132
hemostasis, 131
history of development, 125–6
hypothermia
neuroprotection, 131–2
leukocyte depletion, 134
neurological function monitoring, 136–7
neurological monitoring, 135–7
neuroprotection strategies, 131–7
outcome, 137–8
pathophysiology of hypothermia, 126
pH-stat blood gas management, 132–3
pharmacological neuroprotection, 135
postoperative care, 137
practical considerations, 126–31
preoperative assessment, 126
preservation of organ function, 125
retrograde cerebral perfusion (RCP), 133
re-warming, 130
safe duration of DHCA, 129–30
selective antegrade cerebral perfusion (SACP), 133–4
spinal cord protection, 135
surgical considerations, 128
temperature monitoring, 127–8
desmopressin, 52
bleeding prevention, 51
dextrans, 39
direct thrombin inhibitors, 45
disseminated intravascular coagulation (DIC), 41
$DO_2$. See systemic oxygen delivery
dobutamine, 103
drainage
venous, 57
drug dilution and loss during CPB, 78

# E

ECMO. *See* extracorporeal membrane oxygenation
electrocardiogram (ECG)
 recording during CPB, 64
electrolytes, 76–8
 monitoring, 78–9
 weaning from CPB, 66
emergency cardiopulmonary support (ECPS), 195–6
endothelium
 functions during CPB, 144
endotoxins
 and acute kidney injury, 171
 produced during CPB, 146
enoximone, 103
epicardial pacing, 98–9
equipment
 alarm systems, 20
 arterial and venous saturation monitors, 18–9
 arterial cannulae, 3–5
 arterial line filters, 13–4, 23
 cardioplegia delivery systems, 15–7, 23
 centrifugal pumps, 8
 filters and bubble traps, 13–4
 gas supply system, 13
 hemofilters, 17–8
 history of development, 1
 in-line blood gas analyzers, 18–9
 oxygenators, 10–3, 23
 pumps, 6–8
 reservoirs, 8–9, 23
 roller pumps, 7–8
 suckers and vents, 14–5
 tubing, 1–3, 23
 venous cannulae, 6
extracorporeal membrane oxygenation (ECMO), 176–86
 cannulation, 183
 cardiac ECMO in adults, 179
 differences to CPB, 176
 history of development, 176
 indications, 176–9
 inflammatory response to, 183
 patient management, 183–5
 respiratory ECMO in adults, 177–9
 types of ECMO, 176
 veno-arterial (VA) ECMO, 176–7
 veno-arterial (VA) ECMO cannulation, 183
 veno-arterial (VA) ECMO weaning and decannulation, 185–6
 veno-venous (VV) ECMO, 176–7
 veno-venous (VV) ECMO cannulation, 183
 veno-venous (VV) ECMO weaning and decannulation, 185
extracorporeal membrane oxygenation (ECMO) circuit, 181, 179–83
 anticoagulation, 183
 bridge, 182
 cannulae, 179–81
 heat exchanger, 182
 monitoring, 182
 oxygenators, 182
 pump, 181–2
 safety devices, 182

# F

femoral veins
 cannulation, 6
fibrillatory arrest with hypothermia myocardial protection method, 86–7
fibrinolysis
 after CPB, 52
 in the CPB circuit, 50
fibrinolytic pathway, 144
fibrinolytics, 45
Fick equation, 62
Fick's Law of Diffusion, 10
filters and bubble traps, 13–4
flow rates during CPB, 72
functional mitral regurgitation, 104

# G

gas-exchange mechanisms
 oxygenators, 10–3
gas supply system, 13
gastrointestinal complications of CPB, 148
gelofusine, 39
Gibbon, John, 1, 187
glucose
 serum glucose levels, 77
glucose control

effects on neurological outcome, 157
 weaning from CPB, 77
glycemic control during DHCA, 134

# H

Hartmann's solution, 38
heart-lung transplant, 58
heart transplant, 58
hematocrit (HCT)
 effects of hemodilution, 70–1
hematocrit monitors, 18–9
hemoconcentrators, 17–8
hemodilution, 63
 during DHCA, 132
 metabolic management during CPB, 70–1
hemofilters, 17–8
hemofiltration, 77–8, 146
hemoglobin
 buffering of hydrogen ions, 74
hemoglobin concentration
 weaning from CPB, 94
Hemochron, 47
hemophilia, 51–2
HemoTec ACT, 47
heparin, 42–4
heparin (unfractionated, UFH)
 ACT monitoring, 43
 dosing, 43
 heparin-induced thrombocytopenia (HIT), 43–4
 heparin resistance, 43
 mechanism of anticoagulant action, 42–3
 monitoring, 43
 structure, 42
 use as CPB anticoagulant, 42–4
heparin-bonded circuitry, 146
heparin dosing
 bleeding prevention, 51
heparin-induced platelet activation assay (HIPPA), 44
heparin-induced thrombocytopenia, 43–4
Heparin Management Test (HMT) Cascade analyzer, 47
heparin neutralization, 45–7
 heparinase, 47
 hexadimethrine, 46
 methylene blue, 46–7
 omit neutralization, 47

platelet factor 4 (PF4), 46
protamine, 45–6
heparin rebound, 50
heparin resistance, 43, 61
heparinase, 47
hepatic dysfunction caused by
CPB, 148–9
Hepcon HMS® analyzer, 47
hexadimethrine
heparin neutralization, 46
High-Dose Thrombin Time
(HiTT), 47
hydroxyethyl starch, 39
hyperkalemia, 93
therapy for AKI, 173
hypernatremia
therapy for AKI, 173
hypokalemia, 93
hyponatremia
therapy for AKI, 173
hypoperfusion during CPB, 72
hypothermia, 70
blood gas management, 75
DHCA, 73–4
during CPB, 65, 72–3
effects on hemostasis, 50
pathophysiology, 126
hypothermia (accidental)
re-warming from severe
hypothermia, 190–2
hypoxia and renal damage, 170

**I**

in-line blood gas analysis, 18–9,
78–9
inferior vena cava
cannulation, 6
inflammatory response to
ECMO, 183
inorganic phosphate buffers, 74
inotropic drugs, 94–5
inotropic support
weaning from CPB, 99–100
102–3
integrated method of
cardioplegia administration,
87–9
intra-aortic balloon
counterpulsation, 106–8
complications, 108
description of the IABP, 106
effects on cardiovascular
physiology, 106
IABP placement, 106
management of the IABP
patient, 106–8

intra-aortic balloon pump
(IABP), 105
description, 106
placement, 106
intraoperative ischemia and
physiological management,
156–7
ischemia–reperfusion injury
(IRI), 144–5

**J**

Jehovah's Witness patients, 35,
71

**K**

Kay, Philip, 23
kinin–kallikrein pathway, 143–4

**L**

laboratory investigations, 66
lactate
serum lactate levels, 77, 94
lactated Ringer's solution, 38
latex tubing in the CPB circuit, 3
Lee-White clotting time. *See*
activated clotting time
left atrial (LA) pressure during
CPB, 64
left ventricular assist device
(LVAD), 109
lepirudin, 45
leukocyte depletion, 146–7
during DHCA, 134
levosimendan, 103
liver transplantation
use of extracorporeal
circulation, 193
low-molecular-weight heparin
(LMWH), 44
lung transplantation
use of CPB, 192–3

**M**

magnesium
in cardioplegia solutions,
82, 87
Mg⁺ electrolyte, 77
magnesium level
weaning from CPB, 93, 97
mannitol
in cardioplegia solutions, 87
use in CPB primes, 39–40
mean arterial pressure (MAP),
63–4

mechanical circulatory support,
106–24
history of development, 106
intra-aortic balloon
counterpulsation, 106–8
range of options, 106
ventricular assist devices
(VADs), 108–24
mechanical ventilation
weaning from CPB, 96
metabolic acidosis, 38–9, 72,
74–5
weaning from CPB, 94, 97
metabolic alkalosis, 74–5
metabolic management during
CPB, 70–8
acid-base status, 74–5
alpha-stat management of
blood gas, 75
autologous priming of the
CPB circuit, 71
blood gas managment, 75
causes of metabolic
derangement, 70
DHCA, 73–4
drug dilution and loss, 78
electrolytes, 76–8
flow rates, 72
hemodilution, 70–1
hemofiltration, 77–8
hypoperfusion, 72
hypothermia, 72–4
metabolic effects of CPB
primes, 70–1
monitoring of patient
parameters, 78–9
pH, 74–5
pH-stat management of
blood gas, 75
principles, 70
temperature effects, 72–4
methylene blue
heparin neutralization, 46–7
milrinone, 103
mini-bypass, 20–2
monitoring during CPB, 18–20
Munsch, Christopher, 23
myocardial damage
causes during CPB, 80
postoperative detection
methods, 80
myocardial dysfunction
associated with CPB, 151
myocardial infarction during
CPB, 89
myocardial protection during
CPB, 80–90

myocardial protection during
CPB (*cont.*)
  acute ischemia, 89
  acute MI/arrest cardioplegia,
    89
  alternatives to cardioplegia,
    86–7
  antegrade delivery of
    cardioplegia, 84–5
  aortic root replacement,
    89–90
  cardioplegia delivery systems,
    84
  cardioplegia technique
    modifications, 89–90
  causes of myocardial damage,
    80
  components of cardioplegia
    solutions, 81–4
  definition of cardioplegia,
    80
  evolving myocardial
    infarction, 89
  fibrillatory arrest with
    hypothermia, 86–7
  goals and principles, 80–1
  integrated method
    of cardioplegia
    administration, 87–9
  monitoring cardioplegia
    distribution by
    temperature, 86
  optimum cardioplegia
    technique, 87–9
  postoperative detection of
    myocardial damage, 80
  prevention of septal
    dysfunction, 89
  retrograde delivery of
    cardioplegia, 84–6
  routes of cardioplegia
    delivery, 84–6
  surgical septum, 89
  temperature of the
    cardioplegia solution, 86

**N**

neurocognitive outcomes in
  cardiac surgery, 163–6
neurological complications in
  adult cardiac surgery, 153
neurological function
  monitoring during DHCA,
  136–7
neurological monitoring during
  DHCA, 135–7

neuromuscular blockade
  weaning from CPB, 95
neuroprotection strategies
  during DHCA, 131–7
non-bicarbonate buffers, 74
non-pulsatile (laminar) flow
  during CPB, 8
Normal Saline solution, 38
Normosol solution, 38
NovoSeven (recombinant factor
  VIIa), 52

**O**

oliguria therapy for AKI, 173
OPCAB (off-pump CABG), 47,
  55, 140
  and stroke, 159
  comparison with CPB, 148,
    151
organ damage during CPB,
  140–51
  activation of plasma protease
    pathways, 142–4
  alterations in organ
    perfusion, 148
  comparison with OPCAB,
    151
  complement activation, 143
  contact activation, 142–4
  CPB versus OPCAB, 148
  endotoxins, 146
  fibrinolytic pathway, 144
  gastrointestinal
    complications, 148
  hepatic dysfunction, 148–9
  ischemia–reperfusion injury
    (IRI), 144–5
  myocardial dysfunction,
    151
  pancreatitis, 149–50
  post-CPB ARDS, 150–1
  pulmonary dysfunction,
    150–1
  quality of life after cardiac
    surgery, 151
  role of the endothelium, 144
  role of the kinin–kallikrein
    pathway, 143–4
  SIRS, 146–7
  therapeutic strategies, 146–7
  triggers of organ damage, 140
  *See also* acute kidney injury
    (AKI); cerebral morbidity
    in adult cardiac surgery
oxygen delivery. *See* systemic
  oxygen delivery (DO$_2$)

oxygen demand. *See* systemic
  oxygen demand (VO$_2$)
oxygen-hemoglobin
  dissociation curve, 73
oxygenators, 10–3, 23
oxyhemoglobin
  buffering of hydrogen ions,
    74

**P**

pancreatitis related to CPB,
  149–50
paradoxical intracellular
  acidosis
  weaning from CPB, 97
patient injury or death rates for
  CPB, 28
patient management
  bleeding after CPB, 51–2
patient's notes
  review prior to CPB circuit
    assembly, 25
perfusion during CPB
  pulsatile versus non-pulsatile
    (laminar) flow, 8
perfusion pressure
  effects on neurological
    outcome, 156
perioperative stroke, 157–8
pH
  bicarbonate buffer system, 74
  buffer systems, 74
  during CPB, 74–5
  non-bicarbonate buffers, 74
  normal pH of arterial blood,
    74
pH-stat management of blood
  gas, 75,132–3
pharmacology
  anticoagulation strategies,
    42–45
  interventions for SIRS, 146
  neuroprotection during
    DHCA, 135
phosphate electrolyte, 77
physiological alarms
  CPB monitoring, 20
  re-enabling before weaning
    from CPB, 96
Plasma-Lyte solution, 38
plasma protease pathways
  activation, 142–4
plasma proteins
  buffering capacity, 74
  effects of hemodilution, 71
platelet factor 4 (PF4)

heparin neutralization, 46
platelet function
  abnormalities after CPB, 49–50, 52
  point of care (POC) tests, 48
Platelet Function Analyzer, PFA-100, 48
platelet-rich plasma (PRP) aggregation assay, 44
platelet transfusion, 52
Plateletworks, 48
point-of-care (POC) testing, 47–8
  and transfusion algorithms, 52
post-CPB ARDS, 150–1
potassium
  in cardioplegia solutions, 82, 87
  K+ electrolyte, 76
potassium level
  weaning from CPB, 93
pre-bypass checklist
  design and use of, 25
priming solutions for CPB
  circuits, 36–40
  acceptable hemodilution, 36–7
  association with metabolic acidosis, 38–9
  autologous priming, 37
  avoiding allogenic blood transfusions, 37
  blood-based primes, 37
  children, 36
  colloid-based primes, 39–40
  crystalloid primes, 37–9
  experimental oxygen-carrying solutions, 40
  Hartmann's solution, 38
  infants and neonates, 36
  Lactated Ringer's solution, 38
  mannitol, 39–40
  metabolic effects, 70–1
  Normal Saline solution, 38
  Normosol solution, 38
  Plasma-Lyte solution, 38
  prime volume, 36–7
  purpose of priming solution, 36
  Ringer's solution, 38
  target hematocrit, 36–7
  tonicity of the priming solution, 37–8

types of priming solution, 37–40
Procaine in cardioplegia solutions, 82
protamine
  heparin neutralization, 45–6
protamine dosing
  bleeding prevention, 51
pulmonary artery (PA) pressure during CPB, 64
pulmonary dysfunction associated with CPB, 150–1
pulsatile flow during CPB, 8
pumps used in extracorporeal circuits, 7–8
PVC tubing, 1–3

Q

quality of life after cardiac surgery, 151

R

recombinant factor VIIa (rFVIIa), 52
renal damage. See acute kidney injury (AKI); chronic kidney disease (CKD)
renal replacement therapy for AKI, 173–4
reservoirs, 23
  venous, 8–9
respiratory acidosis, 75
respiratory alkalosis, 75
retrograde cerebral perfusion (RCP), 74
  DHCA, 133
retrograde delivery of cardioplegia, 84–6
right ventricular assist device (RVAD), 109
Ringer's solution, 38
roller pumps, 7–8

S

safety issues
  before, during and after CPB, 25
  rates of patient injury or death, 28
salvaged blood, 9
  suckers and vents, 14–5
  weaning from CPB, 94
  See also cardiotomy suction.

selective antegrade cerebral perfusion (SACP)
  DHCA, 133–4
septal dysfunction after cardiac surgery, 89
serotonin release assay (SRA), 44
silicone rubber tubing in the CPB circuit, 3
SIRS (systemic inflammatory response syndrome), 50, 64, 140–2, 146–7
  and acute kidney injury, 171
sodium in cardioplegia solutions, 82
Sonoclot test, 48
spinal cord
  protection during DHCA, 135
  reducing ischemia during descending aneurysm surgery, 189
St Thomas' Hospital cardioplegia solution, 82
stroke
  and intraoperative physiological management, 156–7
  and OPCAB, 159
  perioperative, 157–8
  risk factors for perioperative stroke, 161–3
  stroke risk in the general population, 161–3
  timing of cardiac surgery-related stroke, 159–60
suckers and vents, 14–5
superior vena cava cannulation, 6
surgical septum, 89
$S_vO_2$ measurement, 78–9
systemic inflammatory response syndrome (SIRS), 50, 64, 140–2, 146–7
  and acute kidney injury, 171
systemic oxygen delivery ($DO_2$)
  blood gas monitoring, 78–9
  influence of temperature, 72–3
  metabolic acidosis, 74–5
systemic oxygen demand ($VO_2$)
  blood gas monitoring, 78–9
  influence of temperature, 72–3
  metabolic acidosis, 74–5
systemic vascular resistance (SVR), 100–1

**T**

temperature
  during CPB, 64–5, 72–3
  effects on neurological
    outcome, 156–7
  influence on blood gas
    management, 75
  weaning from CPB, 92–3
Terumo CDI-500 in-line blood
  gas analyzser, 19
THAM in cardioplegia
  solutions, 82, 87
thoracic aorta, blunt injury, 190
thoracic aortic aneurysms,
  188–9
thoracic aortic dissection,
  187–8
thoracic aortic surgery, 187–90
thrombocytopenia
  after CPB, 52
  heparin-induced (HIT), 43–4
thromboelastography (TEG), 48
  alpha angle, 48
  clot lysis measurement, 48
  K value, 48
  MA (maximum amplitude),
    48
  R value, 48
tissue plasminogen activator
  (tPA), 144
tonicity of a priming solution,
  37–8
total artificial heart (TAH), 106
total circulatory arrest. See deep
  hypothermic circulatory
  arrest (DHCA)
tranexamic acid, 50–1, 131
transfusion algorithms, 52
transesophageal
  echocardiography (TOE)
  during CPB, 65–6
  role in weaning from CPB, 101
trauma care
  use of CPB, 194–5
tromethamine (tris-
  hydroxymethyl
  aminomethane). See THAM
tubing in the CPB circuit, 1–3,
  23
tumor resection
  use of CPB, 193–4

**U**

ultrafilters, 17–8
ultrafiltration, 77–8, 146

uninterruptible power supply
  (UPS), 23
urine volume during CPB, 65

**V**

vasoactive drugs, 94–5, 102–3
vasodilators, 94–5
vasopressors, 94–5, 102–3
venous and arterial oxgyen
  saturation monitors, 18–9
venous blood analysis, 78–9
venous cannulae, 6
venous cannulation and
  drainage, 57–8
  avoiding air entry into the
    system, 58
  cavitation phenomenon, 57
  cavo-atrial cannulation, 58
  connection to the patient,
    57–8
  peripheral venous
    cannulation, 58
  right atrial cannulation,
    57–8
  single cannula approach, 57
  types and sizes of cannulae,
    57
  venous drainage, 57
venous circulation and drainage
  bicaval cannulation, 58
venting the heart, 14–5,
  60–1
  venting methods, 61
  venting the left heart, 60
  venting the right heart,
    60–1
ventricular assist devices
  (VADs), 105, 108–24
  bridge to recovery (BTR),
    110–1
  bridge to transplant (BTT),
    110–1
  categories of potentially
    suitable patients, 111–3
  continuous flow devices, 113
  decision-making process,
    111–3
  description, 109
  destination therapy (DT),
    110–1
  factors affecting output,
    110
  HeartMate II, 116–8
  left ventricular assist device
    (LVAD), 109
  Levitronix CentriMag, 114

long-term care of VAD
    patients, 123–4
  outcomes for patients,
    110–1
  patient management,
    120–3
  perioperative patient
    management, 120–2
  postoperative patient
    management, 122–3

  preoperative patient
    managment, 120
  pulsatile devices (volume
    displacement devices),
    113
  purpose of VADs, 108–9
  right ventricular assist device
    (RVAD), 109
  Thoratec PVAD and IVAD,
    114–6
  types of VAD, 120
  types of VAD systems, 110
  Ventracor VentrAssist, 120
  weaning from CPB with VAD
    support, 122
Verify Now monitoring system,
  48
$VO_2$. See systemic oxygen
  demand
von Willebrand factor (VWF),
  51, 52

**W**

weaning from CPB, 66–7,
  92–105
  adrenaline (epinephrine),
    103
  analgesia, 95
  anesthesia, 95
  arterial blood gases, 97
  assessment and adjustment of
    preload, 99
  assessment of afterload,
    100–1
  assessment of clotting and
    platelet function, 94
  assessment of contractility,
    99–100
  calcium level, 93
  cardiac function assessment,
    95
  chest splinting, 105
  circulating volume, 94
  coagulation, 94
  de-airing the heart, 97

dobutamine, 103
dopamine, 103
electrolytes, 97
enabling physiological
    alarms, 96
enoximone, 103
epicardial pacing, 98–9
events immediately prior
    to, 98
failure to achieve satisfactory
    weaning, 102–5
functional mitral
    regurgitation, 104
glucose control, 93
hemoglobin concentration,
    94
hyperkalemia, 93
hypokalemia, 93
inotropic drugs, 94–5, 96

inotropic support, 99–100,
    102–3
intra-aortic balloon
    counterpulsation, 105
lactate levels, 94
levosimendan, 103
magnesium levels, 93, 97
mechanical support, 104–5
mechanical ventilation, 96
mechanics of separation from
    CPB, 99–101
metabolic acidosis, 94, 97
milrinone, 103
neuromuscular blockade, 95
paradoxical intracellular
    acidosis, 97
potassium level, 93
predicting difficulty, 95–6
preparation, 92–6

re-institution of CPB, 92
re-warming the patient,
    92–3
reversal of anticoagulation,
    94, 101–2
role of TOE, 101
systemic vascular resistance
    (SVR), 100–101
temperature of the patient,
    92–3
use of salvaged blood, 94
vasoactive drugs, 94–5,
    102–3
vasodilators, 94–5
vasopressors, 94–6,
    102–3
ventricular assist devices
    (VADs), 105
with VAD support, 122

Index